Juliane Klein
Transferring Professional Knowledge and Skills

W0038292

Juliane Klein

Transferring Professional Knowledge and Skills

The Case of Central and Eastern European
Migrant Physicians in German Hospitals

Budrich UniPress Ltd.
Opladen • Berlin • Toronto 2016

A CIP catalogue record for this book is available from
Die Deutsche Bibliothek (The German Library)

© 2016 by Budrich UniPress Ltd. Opladen, Berlin & Toronto
www.budrich-unipress.eu

ISBN   **978-3-86388-733-9**
eISBN   978-3-86388-297-6

Das Werk einschließlich aller seiner Teile ist urheberrechtlich geschützt. Jede Verwertung außerhalb der engen Grenzen des Urheberrechtsgesetzes ist ohne Zustimmung des Verlages unzulässig und strafbar. Das gilt insbesondere für Vervielfältigungen, Übersetzungen, Mikroverfilmungen und die Einspeicherung und Verarbeitung in elektronischen Systemen.

Die Deutsche Bibliothek – CIP-Einheitsaufnahme
Ein Titeldatensatz für die Publikation ist bei Der Deutschen Bibliothek erhältlich.

Budrich UniPress Ltd.
Stauffenbergstr. 7. D-51379 Leverkusen Opladen, Germany

86 Delma Drive. Toronto, ON M8W 4P6 Canada
www.budrich-unipress.eu

Jacket illustration by Bettina Lehfeldt, Kleinmachnow –
www.lehfeldtgraphic.de
Editing: Alison Romer, Lancaster, UK
Technical Editing: Anja Borkam, Jena
Printed in Europe on acid-free paper by Books on Demand, Norderstedt

Acknowledgements

This thesis would not have been possible without the help and support of many individuals. First and foremost, I would like to express my sincere gratitude to Prof Karin Gottschall, Prof Steffen Mau and Prof Magdalena Nowicka for their valuable guidance during this PhD project, their scholarly input and constructive feedback. I owe Prof Matthias Wingens many thanks for his assistance with the interview guides, much appreciated advice on several aspects of my thesis and his generous "open door" whenever needed.

I am very grateful for the financial and institutional support of the Bremen International Graduate School of Social Sciences, which provided a favourable environment for conducting this research. I extend my thanks to the German Academic Exchange Service for funding a research stay at the Center of Migration Research of the University of Warsaw. I am deeply indebted to my hosts Paweł Kaczmarczyk and Monika Szulecka for stimulating discussions and to Joanna Nestorowicz for making my stay so convenient.

My deep gratitude goes to the human resource managers, managing and medical directors of the hospitals for agreeing to participate in the interviews. I am particularly thankful to the migrant physicians for their willingness to share their personal stories with me. I admire their endurance, and sincerely hope to do justice to their perceptions and views.

Furthermore, I have to thank Prof Adrian Favell and Prof Jochen Roose for their comments on early versions of my PhD proposal, and Herwig Reiter for precious advice with the analysis of my data. The members of my peer-coaching team, Yuen Fang, Elaheh Daghighi, and Danny Barrantes helped me to not lose my way during the last year of writing up – thank you very much for that! I am very grateful to my dear friends and colleagues for providing comments on earlier drafts of separate chapters, for helping to translate the interview quotes, for proofreading parts of my thesis, and for making the time of my PhD so much more enjoyable. I especially thank Henrike Knappe, Rose Keller, Katharina Bürkin, Anna Hokema, Laura Landorff, Caterina Bonora, Enis Bicer, Eva Loy, Anissa Kirchner, Jasmina Crčić, Melanie Böckmann, and Elizabeth Hirata, my close companion through good times and bad along this PhD journey.

Special thanks go to my father Werner Klein, and my brother Christoph Klein, as well as my grandparents Artur and Irma Lang for always believing in me. I am particularly grateful to my mother, Birgit Klein, for sharing her "real life experience" with the incorporation of migrant physicians in a German hospital, and being behind me throughout these last four years and beyond.

My most heartfelt thanks go to Carl. Thanks for your unlimited support, your tireless encouragement, and for providing the necessary balance!

Table of contents

List of Figures

List of Tables

List of Abbreviations

CEE	Central and Eastern European; Central and Eastern Europe
ECJ	European Court of Justice
EEA	European Economic Area
EU	European Union
EU-2	the Eastern member countries that accessed the EU in 2007, namely Bulgaria and Romania
EU-8	the Eastern member countries that accessed the EU in 2004, namely the Czech Republic, Estonia, Hungary, Latvia, Lithuania, Poland, Slovakia, and Slovenia
FRG	Federal Republic of Germany
GDR	German Democratic Republic
HR	human resource
PCI	problem-centred interview
SHI	statutory health insurance
STEM	science, technology, engineering, and mathematics
SU	Soviet Union
WWII	Second World War

[H]e said, (...) "You're not allowed to do shifts here." – "What do you mean?" – "You've no clue about these things." I was so surprised. Well, for two years I had worked at the cardiology intensive care unit, and this nurse comes saying, "You're not allowed to do shifts. You've no clue."
(CEE migrant physician in German hospital)

1 Introduction

Germany is among those countries of the OECD with the fewest restrictions on labour migration for highly-skilled (OECD, 2013). Given the traditionally restrictive attitude of previous German governments towards immigration, this finding comes as a surprise. For decades, German governments had denied the country's de-facto status as one of the major immigrant countries worldwide. Until the early 2000s, the German governments abode by the ban on recruitment that was implemented in 1973 to terminate the recruitment of labour migrants after the end of the economic growth of the 1950s and 60s. Starting with the unsuccessful Green Card initiative launched in the year 2000, and the following immigration law from 2005, the insight that Germany is dependent on migrants' skilled and highly skilled labour has led to further policy liberalisations. This development is accompanied by the political rhetoric of a culture of welcoming immigrants and appreciating their abilities ("Willkommens- und Anerkennungskultur"). The objective is to represent this paradigm shift to the outside world, and to guide the social interaction with migrants on the part of authorities, employers, and the wider society (BAMF, 2013). In this dissertation I investigate how far this promoted openness, support, and the elicitation of a sense of recognition of the part of the migrant labour force, apply to the case of migrant physicians in German hospitals.

In the last 21 years, the number of foreign physicians in German hospitals has increased by about 24,500 from 10,275 in 1993 to 34,706 in 2014. In 2014 migrant physicians accounted for a share of 9.5% of the overall number of 365,247 physicians practicing medicine in Germany. The biggest group of migrant physicians came from Romania, followed by Greece, Austria, and Poland (Bundesärztekammer, 2015b). In particular, the number of Central and Eastern European (CEE) physicians working in German hospitals has increased dramatically in recent years. From 2011 to 2012, the share of Latvian physicians has increased by 41.7%, followed by Romanian physicians with 41.3%, and Lithuanian physicians with 37.1% (Bundesärztekammer, 2013a). This development is a consequence of an increasing shortage of physicians in Germany that already started in Eastern Germany in the early 2000s (Kopetsch, 2010;

Tuffs, 2003), and has by now also reached rural as well as urban areas in Western Germany, with the exception of major cities such as Hamburg and Berlin (Kovacheva & Grewe, 2015a). The German government and the German medical association addressed this shortage with extensive liberalisations of immigration policies for highly-skilled, in addition to relaxing regulations for controlling access of migrant physicians to the medical profession. Physicians from other member countries of the European Union (EU) particularly benefit from the latter. Based on the EU directive 36/2005/EC on the recognition of professional qualifications, they enjoy an automatic recognition of their credentials in Germany. They are now entitled to the medical license without passing an assessment of equivalence.

Despite these policy changes giving the appearance that all barriers for migrant physicians to practice medicine in Germany have been removed, researchers strongly argue that even if professional qualifications are formally recognised, migrants often encounter major problems complicating their integration into the workplace (Favell, Feldblum, & Smith, 2007; Nohl, Ofner, & Thomsen, 2010). Therefore I argue that the liberalisation of access to the medical profession, while necessary, is far from sufficient in establishing a sustainable integration of migrants into the local workforce. If this problem is not adequately addressed, Germany runs the risk that the potential of the migrant workforce is significantly under-utilised, and the available knowledge and skills are employed in a considerably suboptimal manner. This is a particularly serious concern for Germany as it not only relies on skilled and highly skilled migrants to fill demand, but, irrespective of labour shortages, hosts a large immigrant population. Hence, my major concern in this dissertation is not the question of how to address this shortage of physicians by recruiting personnel from abroad, which indeed is a problematic topic with respect to the issue of brain drain. Instead, my major concern is the assurance of the effective utilisation of migrants' potentials in an increasingly diverse society, and thus, of their equal participation therein. I address this issue by researching the migration and recruitment of CEE migrant physicians to German hospitals. Thereby, I am particularly interested in their incorporation at the workplace, and how they subjectively perceive this situation.

I chose to focus on physicians and the field of medicine, firstly, because health care is a very vital topic and a shortage in this field underlines the urgency of the research problem. Secondly, I chose this field since it is very ambivalent in terms of the transferability of professional qualifications. On the one hand, the academic medical knowledge is very universal. Among EU member countries, medical studies are harmonised so that the credentials are transferable across the EU. On the other hand, medical systems are strongly nationally organised and national medical associations control access to the profession. In Germany, for instance, relevant decisions are made on an even smaller scale, on Laender level, due to the corporate character of the German medical system. Consequently, even within Germany, contents of medical training, as well as standards and requirements might vary, which gives medical practice a very local touch. This local embedding is further emphasised by the kind of work that medical doctors conduct. The necessity to interact not only with colleagues, but also with laypeople such as patients, requires local language skills as well as familiarity with the local culture. Thus, even if formal recognition of professional credentials is guaranteed, the transfer of medical skills and knowledge is a process that is ridden with prerequisites.

Migration of physicians and of the highly-skilled in general, is mainly researched on a large-scale from an economic or political perspective. Researchers focus on trends (García-Pérez, Amaya, & Otero, 2007; Wismar, Maier, Glinos, Dussault, & Figueras, 2011), policies (Hoesch, 2003; Iredale, 1999), and economic benefit (Borchardt, 2006; Fellmer, 2007). As Favell et al. (2007) point out, the topic of integration which is prominently discussed in migration research with regard to so called "ethnic migrants" is hardly made a subject of discussion with regard to highly skilled migrants (see also Ulbricht, 2014). Instead, the highly-skilled are perceived as members of a high-flying elite who easily blend in with the host society, and do not encounter difficulties at the workplace, for instance, in terms of language, different work cultures, or discrimination. Exceptions regarding medical migration are recent qualitative studies, for instance by Wolanik Boström and Öhlander (2012), Ognyanova et al. (2014), or Kovacheva and Grewe (2015b). Nevertheless, the success or ill-success of migration of the highly-skilled is still mainly assessed with regard to the positioning of the migrants at the host country's labour market. Hence, the failure of migration is determined when a mismatch of qualifications occurs. The highly skilled migrants' subjective perception of their migration, however, is hardly considered (exceptions are e.g. Galasińska & Kozłowska, 2009; Nowicka, 2012, 2014). Therefore, empirical evidence on the subjective perception of their work situation is still rare.

In previous research on East-West migration to Germany, CEE migrants are mainly discussed with regard to low-end jobs and in relation to issues of deskilling. Hence, they are very prominent as seasonal workers (Wagner, Fiałkowska, Piechowska, & Łukowski, 2013), carers for the elderly (e.g. Lutz, 2007), and construction workers (Cyrus, 2001). This image has not changed since the accession of the CEE countries to the EU in 2004, and 2007, respectively. While Germany adopted transition regulations in order to postpone granting full freedom of movement to CEE migrants, numerous young and highly-qualified CEE migrants chose to migrate to the UK (Fihel, Kaczmarczyk, & Okólski, 2006). However, being employed at the secondary labour market in the UK, CEE migrants are not perceived by the UK public, nor the German public, in the same way as other highly skilled intra-EU migrants who are seen as simply blending in with society (Favell, 2013). Instead, they are seen as labour migrants doing low-end jobs that natives are not ready to accept

(Favell, 2008b). Accordingly, there is a lack of both studies on post-accession migration to Germany as well as on CEE migrants at Western European primary labour markets.

I address these research gaps and make an original contribution to the investigation of 'new faces of East-West migration' (Favell, 2008b) on the one hand, and to the research of highly-skilled migrants' subjective perception of challenges and barriers in the workplace integration on the other. To this end, I employ an exploratory-qualitative approach. Based on expert interviews with nine human resource (HR) managers and medical directors from seven hospitals located in rural and urban areas of North, East and West Germany, I firstly depict the institutional strategies adopted on the part of the hospital administrations with respect to the recruitment and induction of migrant physicians. Thus, I establish the institutional context of the study. Secondly, I investigate how CEE migrant physicians working in these same German hospitals perceive their situation on-site through 21 problem-centred interviews. The interview participants consist of male and female migrant physicians from CEE EU member countries: Bulgaria, the Czech Republic, Hungary, Latvia, Poland, Romania, and Slovakia. The findings of the migrant physicians' perspective are discussed in the context of the insights gained from the perspective of the HR managers and medical directors. By adopting this approach I provide an encompassing picture of this new form of post-accession East-West migration in the light of liberalised immigration policies and access regulations, as well as pressing staff shortages. The results will be of interest for migration researchers as well as for practitioners in the field.

The thesis is structured as follows. In chapter 2 I provide the background of the study by depicting the development of Germany as a country of immigration (2.1), from the government's denial of the country's status as an immigration country (2.1.1), to the introduction of special mobility rights for citizens of the EU (2.1.2), to its development to one of the most liberal countries for the immigration of highly skilled migrants (2.1.3). Thus, I highlight the drastic changes that have occurred in recent years with regard to the liberalisation of German immigration policies. In the second part of the chapter I further provide the context of the study in terms of the extent of shortage of physicians in German hospitals (2.2.1), discuss explanations thereof, thus giving an insight into the organisation of the German health care system (2.2.2), and explain the legal conditions for migrant doctors to gain access to the German medical license (2.2.3). These elaborations provide an understanding of the structural conditions of the shortage as well as the way in which the growing demand of medical doctors is addressed.

In chapter 3 I discuss previous literature on East-West migration, as well as on the migration and integration of highly skilled migrants in general, and medical migrants in particular. The chapter is organised in a section depicting changes in traditional East-West migration patterns in Europe after the accession of the CEE countries to the EU (3.1), one that deals with institutional and cultural barriers highly skilled migrants can encounter in finding employment, as well as when entering a new workplace abroad (3.2), and one depicting theoretical concepts for capturing the transfer of professional qualifications and skills from one national context to another (3.3). Thus establishing the scientific embedding of my research, I summarise the identified research gaps (3.4), and derive the research questions, as well as the theoretical orientation of the study (3.5).

In chapter 4 I present the research design of the study as well as the methods I employed. I first describe the research interest and the analytical approach of the study (4.1), before depicting the methods of data collection (4.2), namely, the expert interview (4.2.1) and the problem-centred interview (4.2.2). I then explain my sampling strategy (4.3.1) and present the sample of the study (4.3.2), before describing the methods of data analysis I employed for the expert interviews (4.4.1) and for the problem-centred interviews (4.4.2), and closing with reflections on biases and methodological shortcomings (4.5).

In chapter 5 I discuss the findings from the nine expert interviews conducted with HR managers and medical directors of seven German hospitals. The results are presented chronologically, dealing with reasons for why the hospital administrations recruit migrant physicians from CEE (5.1), and in which ways (5.2). I continue with the depiction of the criteria they apply with regard to the recruitment (5.3), the measures they employ for the induction of the migrant physicians during their initial phase in the hospitals (5.4), and their reflections on future prospects on the shortage of physicians and the related recruitment practices (5.5). I end the chapter drawing interim conclusions (5.6).

In chapter 6 I present the findings from the 21 problem-centred interviews with CEE migrant physicians working in the hospitals represented by the HR managers and medical directors, and discuss them in the institutional context derived from the expert interviews. Again, I depict the findings in chronological order of the respondents' migration process starting with the migrant doctors' motivations to migrate (6.1.1) and their migration strategies (6.1.2). These are followed by the challenges and barriers the migrant physicians' encounter on-site (6.2), including issues with the formal recognition of their credentials (6.2.1), communication problems (6.2.2), an unfamiliar work culture (6.2.3), problems in transferring their professional self-concept (6.2.4), conflicts they have with the nurses (6.2.5), as well as incidences of discrimination and symbolic exclusion (6.2.6). Finally, I present their reflections on their migration and their considerations of future plans (6.3), and again end with interim conclusions (6.4).

In chapter 7 I summarise the main findings with regard to the two subsequent research questions, before linking them to answer the general research question of how far the opening accompanying the liberalisations on a structural level is reflected and experienced in the recruitment and incorporation of migrant physicians in German hospitals. I make suggestions for further research based upon the results, and reflect upon caveats of the study. I elaborate on wider implications of the findings for Germany as an immigrant country and end with some final reflections.

2   Setting the Scene

This chapter aims to set the institutional context of the study by introducing the political and sector-specific background of the migration of CEE physicians to Germany. The former deals with the development of German immigration policies (2.1); it describes the period after the end of Second World War (WWII) when its status as country of immigration was denied (2.1.1), the special regulations for intra-EU immigrants (2.1.2), and the implementation of very open policies after admitting to the necessity of immigration after 2005 (2.1.3). Thus, this first sub-chapter explains general attitudes towards immigration prevailing in Germany as well as the legal framework thereof. The second sub-chapter deals with the shortage of medical doctors in the German health care system and the handling of the question of recruitment from abroad (2.2). It depicts the current shortage of physicians regarding its extent in German hospitals (2.2.1), and discusses different explanations thereof (2.2.2). Finally, it outlines the predominant attitude towards the recruitment of migrant physicians in the health care sector providing the context for the legal arrangements of their employment (2.2.3). These depictions serve as a starting point for the case under study.

2.1 The development of German migration policy

2.1.1   "No country of immigration" – immigration policies after 1945[1]

For centuries, Germany, just as the other European countries, was a country of emigration, rather than immigration. It was only after the end of WWII that Germany developed into one of the most important destinations for immigrants worldwide. Nevertheless, for a long time the German government denied Germany's status as a country of immigration (Joppke, 1999, p. 62). Accordingly, there were neither immigration policies implemented to integrate migrants, nor to deal with questions of naturalisation (Heckmann, 2003, p. 51). On the contrary, the goal of measures regarding migration was to restrict immigration and to prevent permanent settlement for an extended period of time.

Due to changed national borders as agreed on by the Allies after the end of WWII, major movements in migration took place, mainly in CEE. Amongst others, millions of displaced persons and refugees from the Eastern territories of the former German Reich, i.e. countries that were allied with, or occupied

---

1   This chapter has been adapted from Klein (2015).

by the Nazi regime, were resettled in Germany (Fassmann & Münz, p. 521f.). Moreover, in the following years, the borders to the Federal Republic of Germany (FRG) were open for German citizens from such Eastern territories, as well as from the German Democratic Republic (GDR) (Hönekopp, 1997, p. 1). However, since all such migrants were of German ancestry, the German government did not regard them as immigrants in the common sense, and therefore, Germany itself not as a country of immigration. Nevertheless, apart from ethnic migrants, labour migrants as well as refugees and asylum seekers were accepted in Germany at certain times during that post-war period.

The first and most significant immigration of non-ethnic German immigrants to Germany after the end of WWII was the arrival of labour migrants during the 1960s. As Germany had experienced a period of economic growth[2] since the 1950s, the German government signed bi-lateral contracts with different countries in the South and South East of Europe in order to recruit labour force from abroad on a large scale. The aim was to meet the increasing demand for low skilled labour. The first country to sign such a contract with Germany was Italy in 1955, followed by Greece and Spain in 1960, Turkey in 1961, Morocco in 1963, Portugal in 1964, Tunisia in 1965 and the former Yugoslavia in 1968 (Birsl, 2003, p. 132). However, the German government insisted on the temporality of these workers' stays and made an effort to prevent their integration. These workers, who were meaningfully referred to as "guest workers", were not provided with German language classes as the proficiency of the local language was not regarded as necessary. Moreover, they were accommodated in special housing outside of common residential areas in order to avoid social contact with local citizens (Hans, 2010, p. 31). Nonetheless, in practice, the concept of guest workers and the planned rotation system was not successful. In spite of having started from the intention of temporary employment, firms soon realised the not least monetary value of workers who were already trained and incorporated. They wanted to keep workers instead of exchanging them for others that had just arrived and were not yet incorporated into the work routine. Moreover, the workers themselves, who were still keen on the idea of a temporary stay, kept postponing their plans to return (Heckmann, 2003). Finally, in the year of the oil crisis in 1973 when unemployment suddenly started to increase in Germany, the German government imposed a ban on recruitment. This meant that guest workers who had lost their jobs, simultaneously lost their permission to work, and thus their residence permits. Guest workers from non-EC countries were not allowed to re-enter Germany once they had left. This was the reason for many Turkish and Yugoslavian workers, who had not lost their jobs, to stay, and to get their spouses and families to join them. Others who became unemployed, even managed to get the permission to

---

2   The period is called "Deutsches Wirtschaftswunder", which literally means "German economic wonder" and approximately lasted from the end of the 1940s to the oil crisis in 1973.

stay with the help of lawsuits referring to universal human rights – in this case, family and liberty rights (Joppke, 1999, p. 64).

Thus, instead of the expected decrease of the foreign population, the number of non-Germans living in Germany grew. This was the time when Germany turned into a de facto country of immigration (Birsl, 2003, p. 133). During the 1980s and 1990s the necessity for integration measures was even recognized on the part of welfare organisations and worker unions. Hence, immigrants got integrated into the German welfare system. Therefore, on the one hand the "relation to the country of immigration" (Heckmann, 2003, p. 52) was reinforced. On the other hand, the government kept denying Germany's status as a country of immigration, thus questioning the immigrants' legitimacy to stay. Measures were even taken to support the non-EU immigrants' voluntary return to their respective home countries (Heckmann, 2003, p. 52), e.g. with the help of "financial incentives and the early pay-out of their state pension funds" (Thränhardt, 2002, p. 349). Nonetheless, large numbers of guest workers stayed in Germany where they and their descendants are still living today.

During the 1980s, ethnic immigration once again became a significant issue when large numbers of ethnic Germans, primarily from Poland, Romania, and the Soviet Union (SU), arrived in Germany. These so called *Aussiedler* were descendants of Germans who had emigrated centuries ago. Due to the definition of the German nation as ethnic community, citizenship regulations were organised according to ius sanguinis meaning that only persons of German descent could hold German citizenship. This rule allowed these *Aussiedler* to immigrate to Germany where they were granted citizenship immediately upon arrival. This resulted in a stark contrast of rights for *Aussiedler* and guest workers: newly arrived Aussiedler were granted comprehensive citizenship rights, whereas immigrants who had been living in Germany for a significant period of time, such as the former guest workers, as well as their descendants, were not allowed to fully participate in society. This was partially changed only recently in the new citizenship law of the year 2000 (see ch. 2.1.3).

Another group of non-ethnic German immigrants that was accepted and arrived in Germany in the time after 1945 was the one of refugees and asylum seekers. This was particularly the case during the 1980s. These immigrants mainly came from Turkey, but also from Romania and Poland. In particular, those who emigrated from the communist countries of the Eastern bloc „were readily accepted" (Hönekopp, 1997, p. 2). By recognising their status as political refugees, Western Germany could prove its ideological superiority to the East and the communist political system (Dietz, 2002, p. 30). However, after the end of the Cold War in 1989, attitudes towards immigrants from Eastern Europe drastically changed. A fear of mass emigration from these countries was promoted by journalists, politicians, as well as researchers in Western Europe. Governments devised scenarios of a new security problem, thus legitimising anti-immigration measures such as increased border control and new restrictions in asylum regulations (Münz, 1996, p. 4; Thränhardt, 1996, p. 210). Besides Austria, Germany felt especially vulnerable due to the immediate vicinity to the former communist countries. This fuelled the perceived threat of Eastern European immigrants flooding the local labour market with cheap labour, and being a burden to the national welfare scheme. This fear was even projected onto the formerly welcomed *Aussiedler*. When their number grew extensively after 1989, housing shortages occurred. This caused "negative feelings" (Thränhardt, 2002, p. 353) among German citizens. As a consequence, restrictions such as language tests, and quotas were introduced to limit their immigration. This limit was reduced several times until it was finally fixed in the year 2000 to 100,000 *Aussiedler* being allowed to immigrate to Germany per year (Dietz, 2002, p. 31).

Thus, the image of CEE immigrants in Germany had changed after the end of the SU. After that period they were perceived as problematic on the part of the German society (Thränhardt, 2002, p. 345), disregarding the urgent need for their labour force, particularly in the construction sector (Martin, 2004). This tension was also reflected in the political rhetoric. In order to overcome this dilemma between rejection and demand, the German government made bilateral agreements with the Polish government as well as the governments of other Eastern European countries in the early 90s. Therefore, the government met its aims of controlling and restricting (illegal) immigration from these countries to Germany and thus avoid permanent settlement of Eastern European immigrants, as well as of meeting the demand for labour (Hönekopp, 1997, p. 8). Just like in the case of the guest workers in the 1960s, work contracts were only issued for temporary stays, and included different forms of work agreements. First of all, there was project-bound work for which subcontracts with German firms were signed. The most important form was seasonal work, mainly in agriculture. Finally, there were guest worker programs set up as exchange programs and targeted at young workers in order to give them the opportunity to gain language skills as well as work experience abroad (ibid., p. 9). These contracts were similarly limited in two key respects: the length of the migrants' stay in Germany, and the kinds of work that migrants were able to carry out. All of these labour migrants were hired for low-end jobs which did not require professional qualifications and which consisted of work that local residents were not ready to accept (Dietz, 2002, p. 39; Hönekopp, 1997, p. 11). In the end, the expected mass emigration from the former communist countries did not occur. Overall, about 4 million CEE citizens left their home countries between 1989 and 1993 (Münz, 1996, p. 4) – compared to 25 million that had been initially discussed (Thränhardt, 1996, p. 210). Instead of settling in Germany permanently, CEE migrants mostly opted for formal and informal short-term stays or circular migration patterns (Wallace & Stola, 2001).

Given this long tradition of protectionist and restrictive attitudes towards immigration, a change in policies could come about only slowly. It was not before 1998 that the, at that time new, German government, a coalition of the Social Democratic Party (SPD) and the Green Party, put an end to the denial of Germany's de facto status as a country of immigration. Labelling Germany as a *country of immigration*, the actual immigration situation in Germany was finally – at least formally – recognized and accepted. This was stressed with the comprehensive change of citizenship law that was passed in 1999 and came into effect in January 2000. It provided the possibility to naturalise for immigrants who had been living in Germany for at least eight years not receiving social security payments, and for their children born in Germany (Heckmann, 2003, p. 55).

It was also this Social Democratic and Green coalition that made a first step towards, once again, opening the German labour market to foreign labour after the ban in 1973. In the year 2000, the government introduced a so-called "Green Card" after the US-American model which was geared at attracting IT-professionals coming to work in Germany (OECD, 2013, p. 70). It was limited to a maximum of five years and thus again aimed to meet current demands rather than offering these migrants a new home. Moreover, with the condition of a maximum income of 51.000€, a high barrier was introduced, limiting the target group for this measure (Tietze, 2008, p. 36). Hence, the initiative turned out not to be the paradigm shift it came along as at first site, but actually represented a continuation of old mind sets restricting immigration (Kolb, 2006) being accompanied by heated debates and populist statements such as "Kinder statt Inder" (children instead of Indians).[3] The IT-professionals mainly attracted by the Green Card were from India, Russia, Belarus, Ukraine and the Baltic States as well as Romania, the Czech Republic and Slovakia (Birsl, 2003, p. 137). However, the respondent rate was lower than expected and the announced boom of "New Technology" failed to appear (ibid., p. 136f.). Hence, this attempt to attract highly-skilled from abroad was not as successful as had been hoped for.

2.1.2 The special case of intra-EU migration

While the attempt to attract highly-skilled from non-EU countries represented a new development in German migration policies, intra-EU migration has been a more common feature following different rules. These rules are rooted in the European Coal and Steel Community (ECSC) which was founded in 1951 and was the predecessor of the EU. While initially the possibility to take up employment abroad was limited to workers in this sector only, the freedom of movement was gradually extended to include further groups of people, as well as in terms of the rights it comprises. The Treaties of Rome in 1957 constituting

---

3   This slogan was used on the part of the conservative party CDU in the election campaign in North Rhine-Westphalia in the year 2000 (see e.g. Martin, 2004, p. 241).

the European Economic Community (EEC) already included the eligibility of all occupational groups to the freedom of movement, apart from those in public service.

Nevertheless, full freedom of movement irrespective of employment was not granted until 1992 when EU citizenship was established in the Maastricht Treaty, making every citizen of an EU member country automatically an EU citizen. EU citizenship allows all citizens of EU member states to settle and take up gainful employment in any other EU country. Additionally, it includes extensive political and social rights for EU citizens working and living in another EU member state. Hence, intra-EU migrants are allowed to vote on the local level, as well as on the European level in any other member state (Koslowski, 2000, p. 121f.; Maas, 2007, p. 50). They enjoy the same rights to social benefits, social housing and tax reliefs as local citizens do. In order to ensure non-discrimination based on nationality with respect to these rights, as well as in the work place, a respective article was adopted in the Treaty on the functioning of the European Union (Vandenbrande et al., 2006, p. 3). All of these regulations broadly removed most bureaucratic barriers and unequal participation rights. Despite these far-reaching rights, including access to welfare benefits, immigration from other EU countries was accepted readily in Germany. "There has never been any important opposition against this process" which was embraced with "enthusiasm for European integration" (Thränhardt, 2002, p. 347).

However, the approval by the German government decreased when the CEE countries of the Czech Republic, Estonia, Hungary, Latvia, Lithuania, Poland, Slovakia, and Slovenia were about to access the EU in 2004 (EU-8), and Bulgaria and Romania in 2007 (EU-2). Similar to the period after the fall of the iron curtain, scholars, journalists, and politicians expected mass immigration from the CEE countries to Germany to occur. This expectation conjured the above mentioned fear of CEE immigrants taking away native peoples' jobs and taking advantage of welfare benefits (Elsner & Zimmermann, 2013, p. 4). The German government implemented transition regulations that had been optionally introduced by the EU. These enabled the *old* member countries to suspend the right to take up employment, as well as access to social welfare for EU-8 immigrants, until the end of April 2011, and until the end of December 2013 for EU-2 immigrants. While three of the member states desisted from restrictions with regard to the accession round in 2004,[4] the other states gradually weakened the restrictions. Apart from Austria, Germany was the only country that exploited the regulations' full run time (Heinen & Pegels, 2006). Hence, although being EU citizens, CEE migrants were not initially granted the same rights that applied to other citizens of EU member countries in Germany. Given the general approval of the free movement of EU citizens,

---

4   UK, Ireland and Sweden.

the full adoption of the transition regulations emphasises not only Germany's restrictive stance towards immigration in general, but towards immigration from CEE in particular.

2.1.3 Paradigm shift towards great openness – immigration policies after 2005

Although scholars had predicted demographic change and labour shortages long before, the German government did not admit this fact and the resulting demand for foreign labour, until the early 2000s. Despite the failure of the Green Card in quantitative terms (s. ch. 2.1.1), the initiative had signalled a basic willingness to recruit the highly-skilled from abroad. Accompanied by discussions about demographic prospects, it fundamentally changed the tone in German politics – on the part of all parties – depicting qualified immigrants as an important resource, and thus turned away from the strict ban on recruitment (SVR 2011: 65). Moreover, it paved the way for a drastic liberalisation of German immigration policies (SVR 2013: 72). This applied particularly to the immigration of highly skilled labour from non-EU countries. A new immigration law from 2005 tremendously facilitated the bureaucratic process of immigration, and reduced the variety of different residence permits to only two (OECD, 2013, p. 74). While the conditions to immigrate, such as a very high minimum income, were still rather restrictive, the main change of the immigration law was the option of a permanent residence permit. This coincided with a change in political rhetoric in which, for the first time, permanent immigration was communicated as political goal (SVR, 2011, p. 66).

However, these changes in legislation did not immediately result in a significant increase in the number of foreign personnel; the shortages of labour continued to grow at the skilled, as well as the highly skilled, level. As a consequence, the German government issued a list of understaffed professions and shortage occupations in 2011, which was extended in 2012. It included occupations in different fields of engineering, IT-specialists and medical doctors. Migrants from these fields required no maximum income, or a lower maximum income. Additionally, the usual labour market check did not apply, meaning that the responsible agency would first check whether there is a German or an EU citizen available to fill the vacancy (OECD, 2013, p. 76).

Moreover, citizens from the *new* accession countries in CEE could benefit from this rule. From 2009 onward, these exceptions from the transition regulations were extended to all university graduates from CEE EU member countries; Germany had initially adopted these exceptions in order to restrict the freedom of movement for CEE citizens until 2011 and 2013. This resulted from a new law that was passed to steer the immigration of the highly-skilled in 2009 ("Arbeitsmigrationssteuerungsgesetz"). This law again decreased the minimum pay that immigrants had to earn in order to take up employment, as well as the minimum investments those had to make who wanted to be self-employed in Germany (SVR, 2013, p. 74). This measure was clearly demand-driven and signified the initiation of a policy of openness towards CEE citizens, although only being applicable to highly-skilled. It allowed immigration only for those who already possessed a work contract, and was not geared towards generally enhancing human capital. Thus, despite opening up, the restrictive attitude remained (ibid.).

The list of occupational and professional fields affected by a shortage became redundant when in August 2012 the German government introduced the EU-wide Blue Card, targeted at university graduates from non-EU countries. Surprisingly, the German government implemented the specifications issued by the EU in a very generous way in three respects. First, the minimum income was again reduced tremendously, particularly with regard to understaffed professions and shortage occupations. Second, the German government renounced from the option of a labour market check. Third, they introduced unlimited access to the German labour market for family members of the persons holding a Blue Card. Fourth, migrant students and foreign academics were given more time to stay in Germany for finding a job signalling a change in orientation towards the individual's human capital. (ibid., p. 75f.).

Hence, German immigration policy has undergone a major shift from its virtual non-existence, ignoring the fact that Germany indeed is a country of immigration and relying on temporary work agreements only, to policies being among the most generous compared to other OECD countries (OECD, 2013, p. 15). This development coincided with the realisation that Germany will have to increasingly rely on permanent immigration vis-á-vis its demographic situation. Although the CEE migrant doctors under study by now enjoy the full freedom of movement and are no longer subject to the regulations for non-EU citizens elaborated on, the restrictive and hesitant attitude they were confronted with might still impact on how they find their way in the German hospitals. Therefore, the question remains in how far this rational orientation displayed in the new immigration rules translates into a genuinely welcoming culture.

2.2 The shortage of physicians in the German health care system

2.2.1 The current shortage of physicians in German hospitals

Health care in Germany is provided by both practices and hospitals. While physicians working in practices deliver most ambulatory general care, specialist care is provided in hospitals (Bidgood, 2013). The number of hospitals has decreased continuously. In 2010, there were 2,064 hospitals, whereas in 1991 there had been 2,411 – a decrease by 14 %. Most of the facilities have closed in the former territory of the GDR, and some have been merged (Bölt & Graf, 2012, p. 113). There also has been a change with regard to the sponsorship of hospitals with an increase of private hospital holders. Between 1991 and 2010, private hospitals have increased from 330 out of 2164 to 575 out of 1758 facilities overall (ibid., p. 115). This amounted to 32.9 %. Another 30.5 % were publically owned and 36.6 % were private non-profit (Bidgood, 2013). Irrespective of the type of ownership, all hospitals that are "accredited in public hospital plans, meaning that they are considered to be necessary to provide equal and nationwide access to hospital care, are eligible for public funds" (Klenk & Pieper, 2013, p. 334). Hence, the owner, i.e. the Land, the private holder, or welfare organisation, respectively, covers the investment costs, whereas sickness funds cover the operating costs.

In 2013, 357,252 doctors practiced medicine in Germany with a proportion of about 3.4 per 1,000 inhabitants. 181,012 of these practiced in hospitals, and 145,933 in private practices (Bundesärztekammer, 2014c). Although their number has continuously increased in recent years, the notion of a shortage of physicians is currently discussed by media, politics, and bodies of the medical profession. This shortage was first apparent in rural areas in the East of Germany in the early 2000s (Tuffs, 2003), when physicians from Eastern Germany left for Western Germany due to better payment (Bundesärztekammer, 2006). Nowadays, rural areas in Western Germany are also affected and the hitherto difference regarding the demand of physicians between East and West Germany has converged (Blum & Löffert, 2010, p. 63f.). Although city clinics, and even university clinics, now also have started to experience shortages (Adler & v. d. Knesebeck, 2011, p. 233) there is still a major divide between urban, congested areas, such as Hamburg and Berlin, that experience very little difficulty in filling their vacancies, and rural, less populated areas (Gerlinger, 2011, p. 13.e11; Kovacheva & Grewe, 2015a, p. 7).

Figure 1 Hospitals affected by shortage of physicians in % from 2006-2013

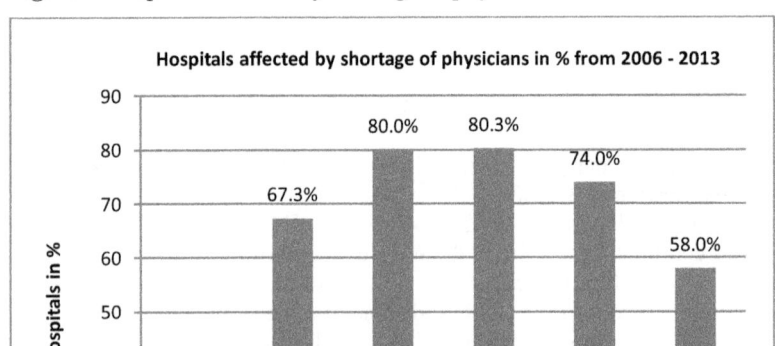

Source: Own diagram based on Blum et. al (2013, p. 31)

However, as illustrated in figure 1, in recent years, the number of hospitals that were affected by staff shortages has decreased. While in 2013, 58% out of all hospitals in Germany had difficulties filling their vacancies with physicians, in the years of 2009 and 2010 approximately 80% of hospitals experienced difficulties (Blum, Löffert, Offermanns, & Steffen, 2013, p. 30f.).

Furthermore, as figure 2 reveals, the average of fulltime medical positions that could not be filled per hospital has decreased. In 2013 the figure was 2.5, which was about 2000 fulltime positions across the whole of Germany being equivalent to 2%. In 2011, 3800 positions had been vacant (ibid., p. 33ff.).

Having a closer look at which hospitals were affected by comparing the number of vacancies announced on the webpage of all German general hospitals in 2012, it is clear that hospitals mainly in the Laender[5] of North Rhine-Westphalia, Baden-Wuerttemberg and Bavaria posted job ads making up 50% of all positions advertised, as shown in figure 3. This is not surprising as these

5   Germany is divided into 16 administrative units called "Bundesländer." Here, the terms "Land" and "Laender", i.e. "federal state" and "federal states" are used to refer to these units.

are the biggest Laender with the highest density of hospitals and accordingly have most positions for medical doctors. Taking into account the overall number of positions for physicians, positions predominantly in the East of Germany were vacant, namely in the Laender of Thuringia (5%), Brandenburg (4.6%), Saxony (3.8%), Mecklenburg-Western Pomerania (3.4%), followed by Saxony-Anhalt and Lower Saxony on equal footing (2.9%) (DKI & medirandum, 2012, p. 13ff.)

Figure 2 Number of vacant medical full-time positions in hospitals with 50 beds and more from 2006-2013

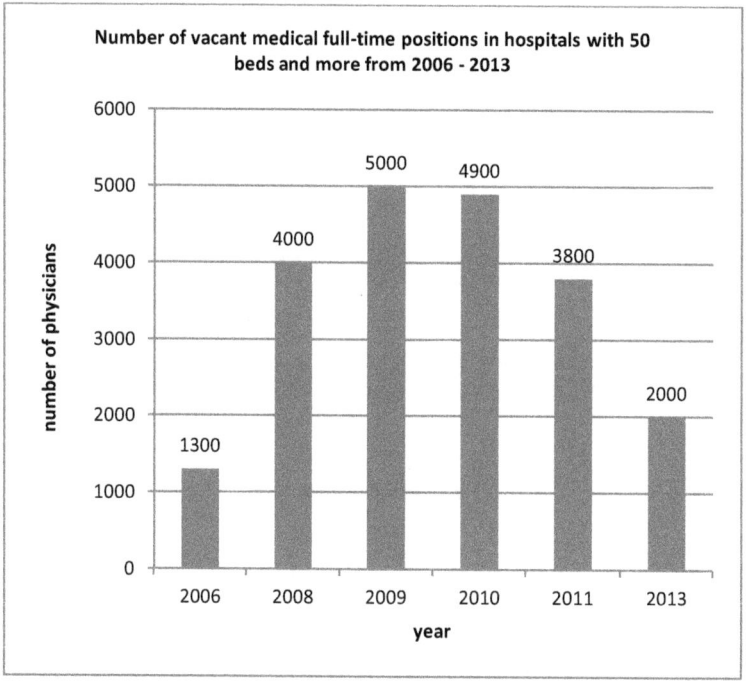

Source: Own diagram based on Blum et al. (2013, p. 33)

With regard to the size of the hospitals[6], medium sized hospitals with 50-299 beds were mainly affected. They posted 44.8% of the job ads (ibid., p. 11), followed by those with 300-599 beds with 29.5%. However, given the actual number of physicians in the hospitals, it shows that smaller hospitals had the highest share of vacancies, namely 7.2% compared to 5.2% in hospitals with

6   Hospital size is measured by beds provided in the hospital. The four different steps are up to 50 beds, 50-299, 300-599 and more than 600 beds.

50-299 beds, and 3.2% and 1.3% in hospitals with 300-599 and 600 beds, respectively (ibid., p. 12).

Figure 3 Job advertisements in relation to medical positions according to the size of the hospital per hundred

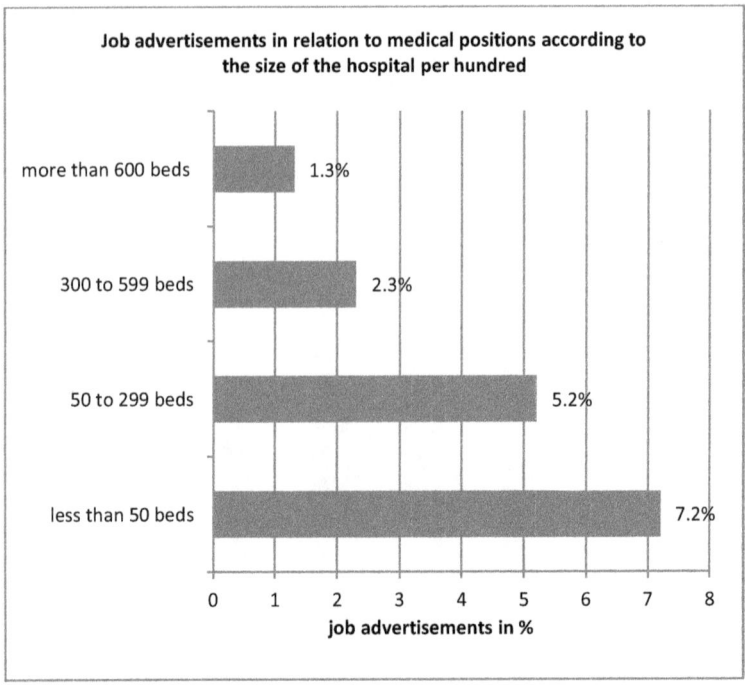

Source: Own diagram based on DKI and medirandum (2012, p.12)

Looking at which hospitals are actually searching with regard to position, it is clear that most positions (50.6%) were vacant for junior physicians in residency[7][8], followed by medical specialists (29.3%). Higher positions were rarely advertised and were thus probably filled internally or with the help of head hunters. As illustrated in figure 4, relative to the number of positions for each group, 3.2% of the specialists' positions and 2.7% of the junior physicians' positions were vacant at the time of enquiry (ibid., p. 6f.).

---

7   In the context of this thesis, the term "residency" neither refers to the place of residence, nor a permit of residence, but means "medical specialist training."

8   In the German hospital system, positions are divided into junior physician in residency, junior physicians having completed residency, i.e. medical specialist, senior physician, and head physician.

Figure 4 Job advertisements in relation to medical positions according to post per hundred

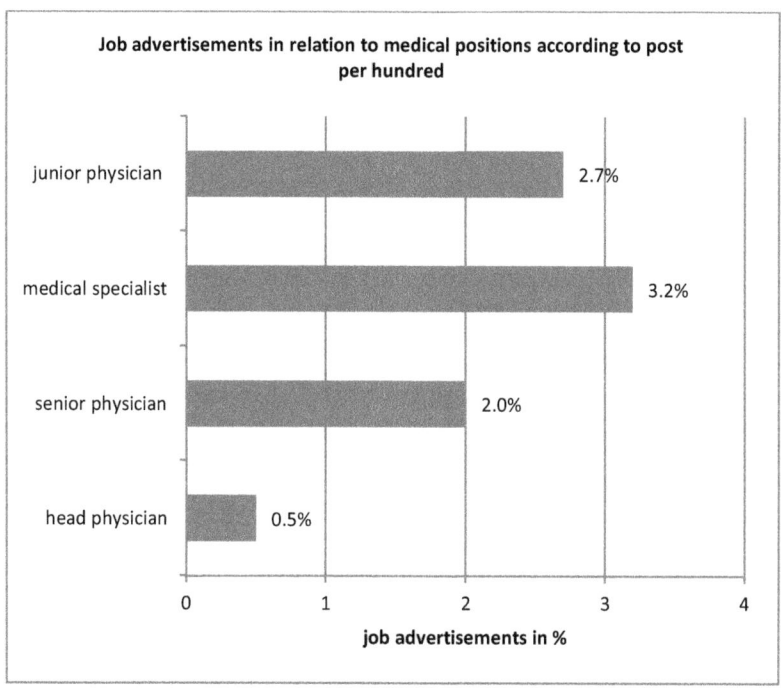

Source: Own diagram based on DKI and medirandum (2012, p. 7)

Junior physicians in residency constitute a large group of physicians in German hospitals. This is because, unless they specialise in a medical field, they are not allowed to open their own practice (Busse & Riesberg, 2004, p. 132). Moreover, unlike in many other countries (Grignon, Owusu, & Sweetman, 2012, p. 7), there is no control of the size of the medical workforce in Germany in terms of a centrally defined cap for residency positions. Already during training, junior physicians are regularly employed and receive a salary which is defined in a collective agreement and increases with every year of training.

Also with regard to the medical field, differences in demand were detected. The fields that were advertised most were unsurprisingly those that are the biggest in terms of the number of positions These are internal medicine, anaesthesia and surgery, making up a share of 34.9%, 13.8% and 13.3% respectively, in the case of junior physicians in residency, and a share of 27.4%, 18.1% and 10.4% in the case of medical specialists (DKI & medirandum, 2012, p. 9f.). Hence, the shortage is very extensive, and affects hospitals in different sizes to different degrees, as well as different groups of physicians.

2.2.2 Explanations for the shortage of physicians

In spite of the figures presented above, the overall number of physicians in Germany has increased during the last years. While in 2009, there were about 325,900 physicians practicing medicine in Germany, in 2013 their number rose to 357,252 (Bundesärztekammer, 2013a). Nevertheless, at the same time there is a significant shortage of physicians in Germany, and a growing demand is predicted for the future. This may at first seem like a paradox, but can be explained plausibly with regard to several developments having taken place in recent years.

The first development is of a demographic nature. Hence, the share of older people in society, and thus among patients, is steadily increasing. Therefore, so is the demand of health care provision, as a high age is shown to be positively correlated with multi-morbidity, i.e. having several chronic diseases at the same time. Thus, more medical staff including physicians is required nowadays, and will be inevitable in the near future (Kopetsch, 2010, p. 131ff.). Additionally, medical progress allows for a wider range of treatments and therapies than ever before. Hence, it increases the lifetime of the individual, leads to an increase of required medical treatments and thus, of required medical doctors to conduct these procedures (ibid., p. 127ff.). Moreover, scientific progress entails an increasing specialisation and hence, differentiation in more medical fields which again requires more physicians (Montgomery in Bundesärztekammer, 2014b).

Another aspect that is discussed within this context is the increasing feminisation of medicine. Thus, the number of female students enrolling at medical schools as well as the number of women practicing medicine is rising. Hence in 2008, 61.3% of all medical students in Germany were female (Kopetsch, 2010, p. 100), and the share of female medical doctors practicing medicine in hospitals increased from 33.76% in 1991 to 43.44% in 2009 (ibid., p. 95). Along with this development, scholars see the reduction of the overall work volume due to an assumed preference for part time work of female physicians as problematic. As a consequence, again an increasing demand of medical doctors is expected (ibid., p. 135f.). However, the wish for a reduction in work time is not exclusive to female physicians, but also applies to male physicians. The reduction of work volume on the part of female physicians was only slightly higher than the reduction of work time by male physicians (Adler & v. d. Knesebeck, 2011, p. 231). Thus, it seems to be a characteristic of young medical doctors – the so called generation Y – to request a better compatibility of family and work, and a better work-life-balance (see also Montgomery in Bundesärztekammer, 2014b).

There are also structural aspects that represent reasons for the increasing demand of physicians in German hospitals. Due to a verdict by the European Court of Justice (ECJ) from September 2003, emergency service had to be considered as working time, even if sleeping facilities were provided for the medical doctors. This change in the Working Time Act additionally intensified the problematic situation. Estimations ranged between 15,000 and 27,000 further positions needed to compensate for the alterations (Hoesch, 2003, p. 109). Further aspects foster the demand. With respect to demographics, not only the average age of the patients is rising; the average age of medical doctors practicing medicine in German hospitals has increased during the last years. While in 1993, the average age of hospital physicians less than 60 years was 38.05, it was 41.25 in 2013. At the same time, the share of physicians under the age of 35 has dramatically decreased from 26.6% in 1993 to 18.0% in 2013 (Bundesärztekammer, 2014a), while the share of physicians aged older than 59 is steadily increasing and has reached 15.6% (Bundesärztekammer, 2014b).

Figure 5 Development of the number of students in human medicine without doctoral students

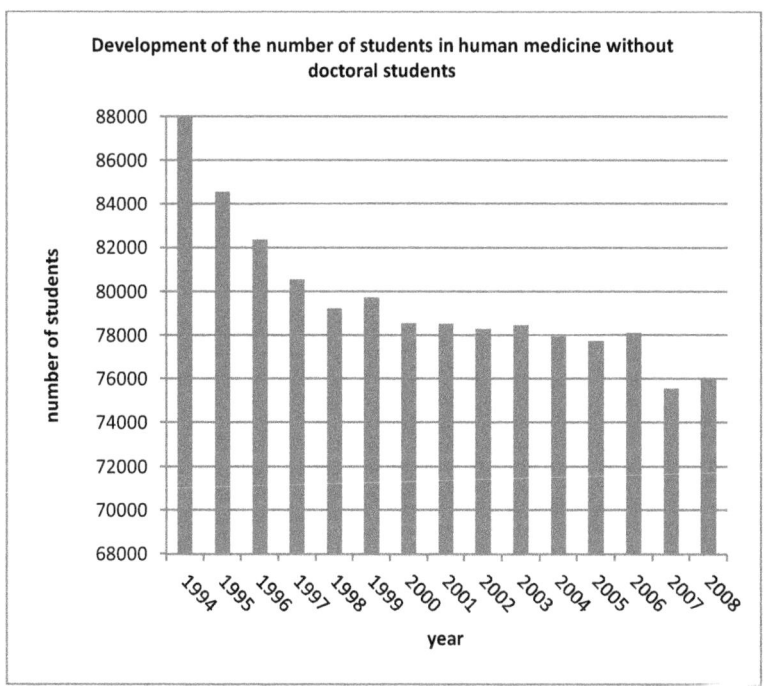

Source: Own diagram based on Kopetsch (2010, p. 36)

However, it is not only older physicians and their upcoming retirement, but also the lack of successors that adds to the shortage of physicians in Germany.

Since a surplus of physicians in the 90s, access to medical studies was restricted by implementing a high numerus clausus[9] limiting the number of medical students. Additionally, in the year 2002, new regulations for the issue of a medical license were implemented that again limited the number of university places (Kopetsch, 2010, p. 32f.). As a consequence, the number of students being enrolled in human medicine decreased in recent years as shown in figure 5.

According to Hoesch (2003, 2012), the reasons for that are inherent in the structure of the German health care system, being significantly influenced by the health insurance act implemented by Bismarck in 1883. Due to the obligation of each citizen to be health insured, but the prohibition for insurance companies to provide physicians and hospitals for their clients, there is a decoupling of health care provision on the one hand, and its financing on the other. Hence, patients can unrestrictedly consume health care that is provided by independent resident doctors who are interested in maximising their profit. Therefore, the medical profession used to be attractive and did not have to worry about staff shortages. However, when in 1992 the Health Care Structure Act ("Gesundheitsstrukturgesetz") was implemented, for the very first time, there was a monetary limit for physicians on how much to spend for health care provision. In reaction to that, the *Association of Statutory Health Insurance Physicians* ("Kassenärztliche Vereinigung") did not reduce the prices, but the capacities for training physicians in order to keep competition low and their income high. Therefore, they lobbied for a decrease in the number of medical students which can be observed since 1992 (ibid., p. 105ff.).

However, apart from the reduced number of students taking up studies in medicine, there is also an increasing drop-out rate of medical students during or after their studies (Hoesch, 2003, p. 104). Hence, in 2002 about 10-13% of medical students in Germany did not finish their studies (Adler & v. d. Knesebeck, 2011, p. 230). Another aspect is the increasing drop-out rate of medical graduates to other professions. While the opening of different professional fields for medical graduates was being encouraged and promoted on the part of employment agencies during the time of the heavy surplus of physicians in the 90s, this now forms one major issue regarding the current shortage of medical doctors in Germany (Hoesch, 2003, p. 104). Hence, medical graduates and physicians opt for different non-curative medical jobs, such as health management, and activities such as consultancy, occupational medicine, and research (Kopetsch, 2010, p. 104).

A final aspect to be mentioned is the growing number of physicians, originally practicing medicine in Germany, who leave in order to work abroad. As illustrated in figure 6, their number increased from 2,249 in 2005 (ibid., p. 122) to 3,035 in 2013 (Bundesärztekammer, 2014b).

9   Access limitation for a certain course of study based on the final grade from high school.

Figure 6 Number of emigrating German physicians from 2005-2013

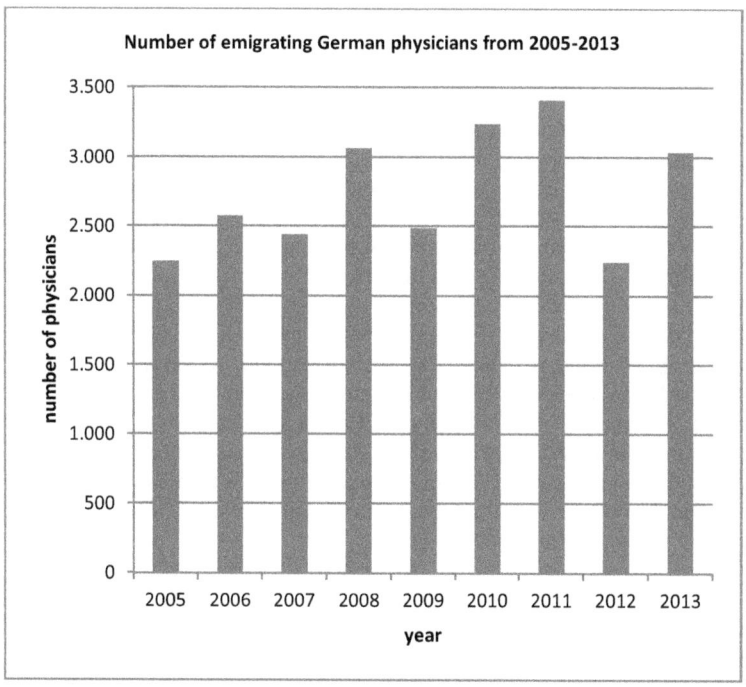

Source: Own diagram based on figures from Kopetsch (2010, p. 122) and Bundesärztekammer (2011, 2012, 2013b, 2014b)

The countries favoured among these physicians emigrating from Germany are mainly the German speaking countries of Switzerland and Austria, followed by the US, and UK (ibid., p. 123). The high drop-out rate of German medical graduates and physicians both to other professions and other countries shows that the medical profession is regarded as less attractive, especially on the part of younger generations. Survey results reveal that the reasons include working conditions, long working hours, and the resulting incompatibility of family and work, leadership culture, payment, lack of incorporation, deficits in the residency training etc. (Adler & v. d. Knesebeck, 2011, p. 230f.). Hence, the German health care system is facing a pressing situation, challenging its hitherto set-up and organisation.

2.2.3 Recruitment from abroad as solution? Attitudes and legal regulations

Reluctance to recruit physicians from abroad

When suggesting strategies of how to cope with this shortage of physicians, the need to present the German medical profession as attractive for young people, and especially women, again by responding to the aspects named above, is most prominent. Accordingly, in-house child care facilities, more flexible working hours, better incorporation measures, and a better structure of residency training are discussed (Bundesärztekammer, 2014b). Interestingly, the recruitment of medical doctors from abroad is not mentioned as a strategy to meet the demand on the part of relevant actors in the field. The intention to solve the problem internally prevails. This corresponds to the observation by Hoesch (2012) that Germany did not immediately react to the increasing demand of physicians with the option of recruitment from abroad, as was the case for other European countries with similar demographic problems such as the UK. Instead, the *German Medical Association* ("Bundesärztekammer") searched for alternative solutions to deal with the shortages. These included attempts to make the medical profession more attractive, particularly for younger generations of physicians, for example with the help of reduced bureaucracy and higher salaries (Finotelli, 2014b, p. 32). Another argument against the recruitment from abroad put forward by *Marburger Bund*, the association representing hospital physicians' interests, was the brain drain caused in the respective countries of origin (ibid., p. 32f.).

Structural issues were also identified as a cause for Germany's reluctance to recruit migrant physicians. Apart from the long tradition of restrictive attitudes and policies with regard to immigration to Germany (see ch. 2.1.1), scholars identify the main motivation of the German medical profession to refrain from this strategy as the preservation of their position of power (Finotelli, 2014a, 2014b; Hoesch, 2012). On the one hand, this refers to the independence of the actors in the field from politics. On the other hand this refers to the corporatist character of the German health care system, being rooted in the set-up of the health care system as introduced with the social security system by Reich Chancellor Otto von Bismarck in 1883. Health services in Germany are mainly funded from social security contributions collected through sickness funds that make up statutory health insurance (SHI) and not from tax. Therefore, the government has little say in the policies of health services and thus limited control (Hoesch, 2012, p. 9). The government sets the legislative framework, but the Laender and municipalities manage its implementation. On this lower level decisions are made concerning health promotion as well as financing and planning in the hospital sector. Corresponding to the principle of corporatism, numerous self-governed civil society organisations participate in this process.

They represent the interests of their members on both a regional and national level (Bidgood, 2013). Crucial and very powerful actors are the *National Association of Statutory Health insurance funds* ("Spitzenverband der gesetzlichen Krankenversicherungen") representing the interests of public sickness funds as well as the *National Association of Statutory Health Insurance Physicians* ("Kassenärztliche Vereinigung") representing the interests of physicians who treat publicly insured patients. They have authority over the regulation of quality standards, the allocation of funding, and decisions about the medical services that insured persons are entitled to (Hoesch, 2012, p. 10).

Apart from membership in the Association of Statutory Insurance for independent physicians, membership in a medical chamber on the Laender level ("Landesärztekammer") is obligatory for every licensed doctor. Due to this compulsory registration, both organisations have large financial resources. Additionally, medical doctors have the ability to organise through the *Marburger Bund* which represents the interests of medical doctors working in hospitals, and the *Hartmann Bund* which represents those being self-employed. Thus, medical doctors have a large influence on health policy and its organisation in Germany, and can shape it in their own interests (ibid., p. 12). In this respect, another argument is the monetary interest of general practitioners and independent medical specialists as outlined above (ch. 2.2.2). After the implementation of the *Health Care Structure Act*, "they are in the first place entrepreneurs and accordingly aim at increasing income return" (ibid., p. 10). Hence, they have a vested interest in avoiding additional competition through migrant doctors.

Liberalisation of regulations controlling access to medical profession for migrant physicians

Nevertheless, in spite of this resistance, the legal situation for migrant physicians has changed tremendously in recent years. To practice medicine in Germany, physicians require a medical license which German graduates from German medical schools receive automatically. Matching the restrictive attitude towards immigration outlined above (ch. 2.1), and the reluctance to recruit physicians from abroad depicted in this chapter, for a long time it was not possible for non-EU physicians to obtain the required medical license. This was the case even if they had studied medicine at a German university (Yamamura, 2009, p. 197). Hence, the reception of the medical license was bound to a person's nationality (Hespeler, 2000, p. 333). The only option to work as a medical doctor in Germany, nonetheless, was a professional permit ("Berufserlaubnis"). This professional permit is temporally limited – mostly to 4 years - and entitles the holder to practice medicine only in the Land in which the permit is obtained. Moreover, it does not allow physicians to open their own practice. To this end, a medical license is required. Such a license entitles a physician to indefinitely exercise their profession in a hospital or in their own medical practice in all Laender in Germany (BAMF, 2011, p. 24). Based on this procedure, which is frequently legitimised with the need to protect German medical standards (Finotelli, 2014a, p. 503; Hoesch, 2012, p. 6), migrant physicians could be excluded, for example, from the profitable option to open a medical practice. At the same time, they could be specifically appointed in order to meet upcoming demands (Finotelli, 2014b, p. 35).

EU-physicians, however, were entitled to obtain this medical license. Since 2007 when the EU directive 2005/36/EC of the European Parliament and the European Council on the recognition of professional qualifications came into effect, their qualifications are automatically recognised if they are gained by an EU citizen in an EU country after the accession of this country to the EU. Accordingly, if medical studies were finished before the EU accession of the country the studies were completed in, the respective physician has to provide a certificate of conformity stating that the acquired qualifications equal those listed in the directive. This confirmation is issued by the country where the studies were completed and entitles the physician to receive the medical license and thus, to take up residency in Germany (BAMF, 2011, p. 58). However, the medical license (and the professional permit, respectively) issued by the health department of the Land in which the physician wants to work only represents a first step towards the recognition of their professional qualifications. This further requires the recognition of their medical specialisation on the part of the responsible chamber (ibid., p. 24), again emphasising the influence on the part of the medical professional body. Medical specialists from other EU countries can also obtain a medical license. However, medical specialists from an Eastern member state have to provide a certificate of conformity and prove a certain minimum duration of professional practice as a medical specialist. Furthermore, the medical associations only recognise individual years of residency training in another EU country that has been commenced but not completed. In that case, the responsible medical association in the respective Land checks which aspects of the residency can be transferred. Migrant physicians have to complete missing aspects regarding time or content of the training in Germany before taking the specialist examination. Since 2010, EU citizens are no longer entitled to apply for a temporary work permit (ibid., p. 59). However, when the acknowledgement procedure lasts for an extended period of time, a temporary work permit can be obtained in order to bridge the waiting time, as the process of issuing the medical license can last several months (ibid., p. 54). In the course of these developments, the strict regulations for non-EU doctors were also liberalised, which occurred as a consequence of the growing demand for medical doctors in Germany (Schiller, 2010, p. 79f.). Additionally, the general paradigm shift in immigration policies alleviating barriers to the German labour market for highly skilled migrants might have contributed to these changes (Finotelli, 2014b, p. 36). Based on the new recognition law ("Anerkennungsgesetz") which came into force in 2012, the nationality of an applicant was no longer the ground on which medical licenses were issued, but the country in which the medical degree was obtained (ibid.).

A crucial prerequisite to receive the medical license is German language proficiency as stated in the Federal Medical Code ("Bundesärzteordnung"). "However, the law does not exactly define, which level of language is meant nor how such knowledge is to be assessed" (Finotelli, 2014b, p. 39). Initially, the chambers informally agreed on a level of B2 of the European Framework of Reference (intermediate) which was to be assessed by the responsible health departments on-site. In most cases, the submission of a certificate confirming the desired level sufficed. However, as repeatedly insufficient language proficiency on the part of migrant physicians was criticised, the chambers in Rhineland-Palatinate and North Rhine-Westphalia took over the responsibility for performing a language test from the responsible Health Departments in 2012 and 2014, respectively. In these tests, migrant physicians are asked to write a discharge letter and to simulate a doctor-patient conversation (Hillienhof & Hibbeler, 2014). In 2014, the chambers agreed on the requirement of additional knowledge of medical terminology at the level C1 (advanced). Nonetheless, again these agreements remained informal. The application is not yet compulsory, and has to be decided upon at the Laender level (n.n., 2014). Finotelli (2014a, p. 511) found the hesitation in this respect to be based on the fear of potentially deterring migrant physicians with overly demanding language requirements, and criticised the slow action in tackling this important problem.

Increase of migrant physicians in Germany

Even after these liberalisations the recruitment of migrant physicians was not mentioned as an explanation for decreasing shares of vacancies or decreasing numbers of hospitals affected (see e.g. Blum et al., 2013) until 2014 when the statistics from the year 2014 were presented by the German medical association. For the first time a slight discharge of the pressing situation due to the inflow of migrant physicians was stated (Bundesärztekammer, 2015a). This remarkable lack of interest vis-à-vis the dramatic shortage of physicians can also be observed with regard to the deficiency of statistical information on migrant medical doctors in Germany; the only information available is the physicians' nationality.

Irrespective of the inconsistencies in the attitude of actors in the German medical field towards the recruitment of migrant physicians, their number has increased tremendously in recent years. As figure 7 illustrates, in 1993 10,275 foreign physicians have been practicing medicine in Germany, while in 2014 it has been 34,706. Hence, their overall number increased by almost 24,500 within the last 11 years.

Figure 7 Development of number of foreign physicians practicing medicine in Germany

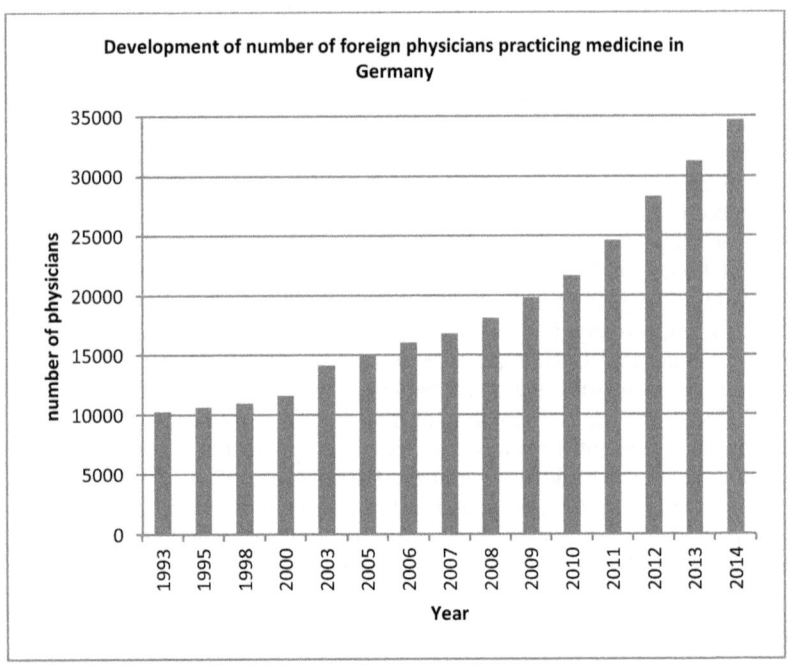

Source: Own diagram based on Bundesärztekammer (2015b)

In 2014, foreign physicians accounted for a share of 9.5% of the overall number of practicing physicians in Germany, i.e. 365,247. Compared to the previous year, the number of foreign physicians has increased by 11.1%. The number of the physicians from other EU member countries has increased most between 2013 and 2014, namely by 1,692, i.e. 8.5%. Romanian physicians form the biggest group with a number of 3,857, before the traditionally strong groups from Greece and Austria consisting of 3,011 and 2,695 physicians, respectively, and 1,936 Polish physicians (Bundesärztekammer, 2015a). The number of CEE physicians strongly increased in particularly in the years 2011 and 2012. Since I started the collection of interview data in 2012, I here present the numbers of this year. In 2012 20,310 physicians practicing medicine in Germany did not hold the German citizenship, and 16,027 of them came from other EU member countries (Bundesärztekammer, 2013a). As table 1 shows, of those EU physicians practicing in hospitals, already in 2012 the biggest group came from Romania, followed by Greece, Austria, and Poland. However, the increase compared to the previous year was highest among Latvian (41.7%), Romanian (41.3%), Lithuanian (37.1%), and Hungarian (34.2%) physicians compared to a very low increase, for instance, on the part of Austrian physicians (0.2%) revealing a clear migration trend from the CEE countries.

Table 1 EU physicians practicing medicine in German hospitals in 2012

Country of origin	Practicing in German hospitals	Change to previous year in %
European Union	12,626	17.7
thereof		
Austria	1,642	0.2
Belgium	158	12.9
Bulgaria	885	18.5
Cyprus	118	31.1
Czech Republic	609	16.7
Denmark	22	-4.3
Estonia	33	32.0
Finland	35	0.0
France	162	5.9
Greece	1,772	18.1
Hungary	919	34.2
Ireland	23	21.1
Italy	583	5.4
Latvia	119	41.7
Lithuania	196	37.1
Luxemburg	161	8.1
Malta	4	0.0
Netherlands	317	6.4
Poland	1,212	6.8
Portugal	63	6.8
Romania	2,399	41.3
Sweden	45	2.3
Slovakia	779	20.8
Slovenia	27	17.4
Spain	225	12.5
United Kingdom	118	3.5

Source: Own table based on Bundesärztekammer (2013b)

In summary, the restrictive attitude as well as the legal opening for highly skilled immigrants characterising the development of German immigration

41

policies vis-á-vis an increasing demand for highly skilled migrants is mirrored in the stance towards, and way of coping with, the recruitment of migrant physicians on the part of the German medical association, as well as other actors involved. Based on the growing demand for physicians due to demographic as well as structural developments, the medical association slowly liberalised the accession regulations for migrant physicians. The shift from highly restrictive to more open policies is therefore clearly demand-driven. This measure shows its effect particularly on the part of CEE migrant physicians, who after the accession of their countries to the EU enjoy extensive rights in terms of freedom of movement as well as the formal recognition of professional qualifications across the EU. Accordingly, their number has increased significantly in German hospitals in recent years.

3   East-West, intra-EU, and highly skilled – integrating different strands of migration research

The aim of this chapter is to review the crucial literature for the investigation of recent migration of physicians from CEE EU member countries to Germany. The purpose of the study at hand is to assess their professional integration in German hospitals in order to find out about potential barriers and challenges they encounter on-site. To this end, the research speaks to three different bodies of migration literature, namely: research on post-accession East-West migration in Europe, migration of the highly-skilled in general, and migration of physicians in particular. These strands have so far been discussed separately seeing the migrants with regard to a certain character trait only, e.g. as CEE migrants, i.e. a specific ethnic group entering local labour markets, or in their capacity as physicians, i.e. in terms of their high qualifications, and thus as valuable contributors to Western welfare sates (for the case of Germany see: Thränhardt, 2002). In line with Favell et al. (2007), who argue that the general classification of migrants into such groups creates a one-dimensional picture of global migrants that does not reflect their real life experiences, I aim to link these different branches of migration literature.

Favell et al.'s (2007) proposed research agenda focusing on "the human face"[10] of migration by focusing on the individual migrant instead of relying on "aggregate data and structural logic" (ibid., p. 15), is particularly informative. They propose that highly skilled migrants in unfettered migration spaces are ideal research subjects, since they are regarded most likely to move voluntarily, and assumed to be least likely to encounter barriers such as exclusion or discrimination. This applies, for example, to EU citizens holding comprehensive mobility rights within the EU (see ch. 2.1.2), and thus lending themselves to investigate the boundaries of an allegedly ever more liberal global mobility. Favell and colleagues (2007) discuss five points of criticism of previous migration research, namely, the dichotomisation of migrants into groups of 'skilled' versus 'unskilled', and 'ethnic' versus 'highly skilled' migrants (1); the assumption that highly skilled migrants are always welcomed on the part of the host country and therefore do not encounter institutional barriers abroad (2); the appropriation of highly skilled migration under the topic of brain drain (3); the assumption that short-term mobility patterns are free from state control (4); and the approach to highly skilled migration from a human capital perspective (5). Drawing on these considerations, I use three critical points Favell and colleagues (2007) raise that are relevant to my study to found my argument through the migration research literature, specifically the criticism of the di-

---

10   See Favell et al. (2008) for a later version.

chotomisation between different groups of migrants, the criticism of the assumption that highly skilled migrants do not encounter institutional barriers, and the criticism of the application of the human capital approach to explain the transfer of professional qualifications. I employ these three points as a lens to review the relevant literature informing my research.

To this end, I draw on Favell et al.'s (2007) criticism of the polarised discussion of distinct migrant groups by referring to the previous depiction of CEE migrants in Europe, and exploring diverse migration patterns in post-accession East-West migration (3.1). I then bring together the second and third point of criticism launched at the human capital approach, in order to highlight the false assumption that highly-skilled migrants do not meet incorporation problems in the work place. Rather, an institutional perspective encompasses employment issues pertaining to the non-accreditation of professional qualifications. Therefore, I discuss empirical findings on various barriers in obtaining formal recognition and adequate positioning as well as barriers to induction at the workplace in the second sub-chapter (3.2). In the third sub-chapter, I address conceptual approaches posing an alternative to the human capital approach (3.3). Based on this literature review, I then identify the research gaps I address with my study in a fourth sub-chapter (3.4), before ending with a fifth sub-chapter in which I present the research questions of the study (3.5).

3.1 Changing patterns of (East-West) migration in Europe: dissolving dichotomies and exploring diversity

One point of criticism raised by Favell et al. (2007) and other scholars in the field (e.g. King, 2002) is the dichotomisation of 'unskilled'/'skilled' migrants and of 'ethnic'/'highly skilled' migrants. They argue that the classification of migrants in this way masks the actual variation within migrant groups and generates a one-dimensional picture. 'Ethnic migrants' for instance are seen as an underprivileged group struggling with barriers and inequalities, whereas highly skilled migrants are regarded as elites existing outside the constraints of social structure. Both groups resemble opposite ends of a continuum that disregards the vast majority of migrants that span the void. This conception does justice neither to the heterogeneity of migrants and their socio-economic background (e.g. their education, level of skills, and the occupational positions they held before migration), nor to their migration motivations and the employed variety of migration strategies. Consequently, scholars call for the dissolution of these classifications and towards the notion of 'middling migrants' (Conradson & Latham, 2005; Ryan, Klekowski Von Koppenfels, & Mulholland, 2015).

The 'middling migrant' in intra-EU migration research

A research strand, in which the 'middling migrant' is most prominent, is intra-EU migration. The liberalisation of migration policies and the establishment of far reaching mobility rights extended to every EU citizen, irrespective of employment, allowed the possibility to stay and work in other EU member states (see ch. 2.1.2). In order to stress these bureaucratic facilitations, scholars describe intra-EU migration as international turning into internal migration referring to the respective migrants as international or EU *movers* (King, 2002, p. 92; Recchi, 2008, p. 71). Additionally, the encompassing suspension of barriers allows for short-term stays since no visa or work permissions are required complicating such undertaking. In this respect, the term 'migration' is replaced by the term '(spatial) mobility' (King, 2002) that stresses the back and forth movement between home and host country (Cyrus, 2000). Thus, various forms of migration and mobility are accessible to all EU citizens, and are not reserved for high-achieving professionals.

In line with these considerations, empirical studies show that intra-EU migration is neither a phenomenon of high-achieving elites, nor mainly embarked on by stranded individuals migrating for material ends. As part of the prominent PIONEUR study surveying data on migrants from and to Germany, the UK, France, Italy, and Spain (Recchi & Favell, 2009), Braun and Arsene (2009), but also authors of smaller scale quantitative and qualitative empirical studies found that intra-EU migrants are mainly middle-class university graduates (e.g. Favell, 2008a; Verwiebe, 2004). However, they encompass not only movers in employable age, but include groups such as students (e.g. Carlson, 2013; King & Ruiz-Gelices, 2003) and pensioners (e.g. Gustafson, 2002; King, Warnes, & Williams, 1998). Correspondingly, migration motives of EU movers are also diverse. While work-related reasons were the dominant migration motives in Europe from the 1950s to the early 1970s, more recent intra-EU migration points to the surge of family and other social reasons, reasons related to education and language learning, or amenity migration; i.e. migration to idyllic landscapes and a warmer climate (King, 2002; Mau & Verwiebe, 2010; Santacreu, Baldoni, & Albert, 2009; Verwiebe, Wiesböck, & Teitzer, 2014).

Hence, in studies on intra-EU migration, traditional classifications of migrants and their migration motives do not apply. Instead, the diversity of groups of migrants and migration patterns find their expression. At the same time, there is the risk to create a new category, namely the one of intra-EU migrants. However, the studies presented above, do not yet include the Eastern member states that accessed the EU in 2004 and 2007, respectively. Research on post-accession East-West migration within the EU proves such a category to be too general, since this migration flow differs not only with regard to previous intra-EU migration, but also with regard to pre accession East-West migration. Additionally, CEE post-accession migration is diverse in itself.

The perception of CEE EU movers

In spite of the EU membership of the CEE countries since 2004 and 2007 respectively, CEE migrants within the EU are not primarily perceived as EU movers like their Western counterparts, but rather as economic migrants seeking employment in the labour markets of the older EU member states. They are classified as a specific ethnic group that is conceived as a threat on the one hand, and as cheap labour force doing work natives would not, on the other (Favell, 2008b). With regard to the former, their post-accession migration is particularly discussed in primarily quantitative studies and against the background of their impact on the labour market, for example in Germany (e.g. Dietz, 2007; Kaczmarczyk, 2007). Regarding the latter, evidence mainly stems from qualitative studies, such as MacKenzie and Forde (2009), on the numerically stronger post-accession migration from the CEE member countries to the UK. They conducted in-depth interviews in a UK based company in the low-skilled sector with the managing director, the general manager, and the training manager, as well as with 10 out of the 40 employees. The latter came from Poland, Latvia, Lithuania, Estonia, but also Portugal and Albania. The employers stated to hire migrant work force due to their good work ethics and because they were willing to work hard, follow the instructions, and work long hours without complaining (ibid., p. 150). Hence, these migrants are stigmatised as a hard working group that is willing to work under poor conditions which distinguishes them from local and other (Western) EU workers.

This unequal status of CEE migrants was also identified by Ciupijus (2011) who analysed the rights granted to EU-8 migrants in the UK and the migrants' labour market experiences. He pointed to the contradiction between EU citizenship granting spatial mobility on the one, and the employment in low-end jobs under poor labour market conditions reflecting downward mobility on the other hand. He concluded that instead of creating a common market with more and better jobs for all EU citizens as strived for by the EU, a dual labour market was produced as Piore (1979) had identified for the guest worker schemes, with a confinement of CEE migrants to the secondary labour market segment. This status difference was found to be even more pronounced in the case of EU-2 migrants in the UK. Other than migrants of the previous Eastern accession round, Romanian and Bulgarian migrants had to initially face transition regulations for taking up work in the UK which brought them into an even weaker position since their access to the labour market was restricted to certain low- and un-skilled jobs, e.g. agricultural work (Fox, Moroşanu, & Szilassy, 2012). This was further illustrated by Ivancheva (2007) in her ethnographic study on Romanian and Bulgarian students who came to the UK as seasonal workers in agriculture experiencing poor conditions and exploitation on-site. She concluded that this transition regulation "creates a 'second-hand' EU citizenship" (ibid., p. 116, original emphasis).

While the connotation with which post-accession CEE migrants were per-ceived in the UK also changed from 'welcome cheap labour' to 'threat to local jobs' after recession, the overall perception of them as different from Western EU movers persists. As Favell (2013) stated, the former have not managed to "become 'invisible Europeans' like the others" (ibid., p. 57), but are instead still or again perceived as regular immigrants threatening the Western EU member states' labour markets and welfare benefits in financially difficult times. Therefore, with respect to the acceptance and perception of CEE mi-grants by the Western host countries, there are major differences between CEE and Western European EU movers.

Perpetuating old classifications in CEE post-accession migration to Germany

The polarisation of 'low skilled' and 'highly skilled' migrants is reflected also in empirical research on CEE migrants in Germany, which concentrates on migrants in low-end jobs. This is still the case after the accession of the CEE countries to the EU (see e.g. Wagner et al., 2013). Although the German gov-ernment adopted the transition regulations in order to postpone the full freedom of movement to CEE migrants, these were already suspended for highly skilled migrants in 2009 (see ch. 2.1.2). Despite this fact, CEE migrants in highly skilled jobs remained invisible in Germany. Nonetheless, CEE highly skilled migrants working in appropriate occupations in Germany do exist, albeit in lower numbers. For instance, the presence of CEE medical doctors practicing in German hospitals is not a new phenomenon, but began in the Eastern part of the country in the early 2000s (Kopetsch, 2010). Yet, they appear only in supply-side statistics of studies on how to manage their immigration (Bor-chardt, 2006; Fellmer, 2007), rather than in qualitative studies exploring the conditions and circumstances thereof. Hence, while the migration of CEE mi-grants working in low-end jobs in Germany is given a 'human face' (Cyrus, 2001; Glorius, 2007), this does not apply to the, certainly numerically smaller, group of CEE migrants holding positions at the upper segment of the labour market.

Additionally, the visibility of CEE immigrants in low-end jobs in Germany is primarily a consequence of the focus on gender-typical fields in the domestic sector. For men this is maintenance and gardening (Palenga-Möllenbeck, 2013a, 2013b), while women engage mainly as carers for the elderly in private households (Gottschall & Schwarzkopf, 2010; Lutz, 2007; Lutz & Palenga-Möllenbeck, 2010). Particularly the latter is classified as work with little social esteem that locals do not accept as employment. The fact that migrant workers enable German women to paid employment and thus to a self-determined life at the cost of less-privileged women (Roig, 2014), further strengthens the im-age of them not possessing any skills (see also: Kofman, 2000; Kofman,

Phizacklea, Raghuram, & Sales, 2000). Accordingly, the frequently chosen focus on women migrants working in the domestic and caring sector diminishes their visibility as skilled or highly skilled migrants (Kofman & Raghuram, 2010). The limitation in research on female migrants to gender-specific occupations, additionally neglects potential gender differences within, for instance, a particular group of migrant professionals (Favell et al., 2007). Although Kofman and Raghuram (2010) argue that due to skill shortages a gender-balance has been established among certain highly skilled migrant groups such as physicians, the question remains whether their induction at the workplace follows the same patterns as the one of their male counterparts. Consequently, with regard to CEE migrants in Germany, there is not only a lack of visibility of highly skilled migrants in the upper segment of labour market in general, but particularly also a lack of visibility of *female* highly skilled migrants and their migration and integration patterns.

Breaking up old patterns in CEE post-accession migration to the UK

So far, post-accession CEE migration to Germany has been discussed as not significantly different from its pre-accession counterpart in terms of who migrates and how (Kaczmarczyk, 2011). Therefore, research on post-accession migration from CEE has mainly focussed on UK as a destination country, providing important insights that I can draw on, since the visibility of CEE highly skilled migrants, post-accession migration to the UK has diversified in several respects (see e.g. Black, Engbersen, Okólski, & Pantiru, 2010; Burrell, 2010; Glorius, Grabowska-Lusinska, & Kuvik, 2013) and softened the sharp low skills/high skills-divide.

Major aspects stressing this claim are firstly, the migrants' high qualifications since most of them are university graduates (Fihel et al., 2006), and secondly, the fact that their migration is discussed in terms of highly skilled migrants. Thus, they are regarded as such in spite of the fact that they largely experience mismatches of qualification and forms of de-skilling, because they are employed in lower sectors of the local labour market (agriculture, food processing, and hospitality), and are working under very poor conditions, long working hours and low income (Clark & Drinkwater, 2008; Currie, 2007; Drinkwater, Eade, & Garapich, 2009). Hence, there is a softening of the polarisation between precarious low skilled and unfettered highly skilled migration with regard to this specific group. Although this does not increase their visibility in the upper sections of the host country's labour market, it does counteract the image of CEE migrants not possessing high skills and qualifications. The scholarly search for the barriers causing this mismatch of qualifications highlights an increasing acceptance of highly skilled migrants encountering difficulties in finding their way abroad further dissolving the common image of mobile elite professionals.

Migration motives

Inter alia, migration motives, strategies, and forms were identified as contributing to the mismatches CEE migrants experienced in the UK. Hence, while among others Engbersen and Snel (2013) regard CEE post-accession migration still as mainly economically driven, other scholars researching the migration motives of post-accession Eastern migrants mainly to the UK softened this claim. Krisjane, Berzins, & Apsite (2013) and Pietka, Clark, & Canton (2013) focussing on young migrants from Latvia and Poland to the UK, found with the help of in-depth interviews that they indeed migrated to find work in the UK, but primarily not to earn more money, but with the purpose of improving their English language skills, gaining (work) experience abroad, and experiencing a different life style. Thus, also post-materialist ends played a role similar to the ones identified for Western EU movers. This shows that migration motives of CEE migrants have diversified, but also that within this group various reasons for emigration apply, again stressing the inadequacy of broad categories.

Migration strategies

This diversity is again mirrored in the employed migration strategies. Engbersen and Snel (2013) identify post-accession migrants to rely on more individual strategies and to be less embedded in family relations than they used to be prior to EU accession. This is confirmed by Ryan and colleagues (2008) who found in in-depth interviews with Polish migrants to the UK that while the traditional ethnic migration networks in the host countries are still in place, they lost in significance at the same time. Due to facilitated ways of communication, it is easier for young migrants to build new networks and to quickly activate formerly established ones. Additionally, migrants increasingly rely on agencies taking care of job search, flat hunting etc. in the host country, and hence institutionalised networks. However, with the help of a mixed methods design including survey data, semi structured, in-depth interviews with EU-8 migrants and interviews with key actors, Sporton (2013) adds that even when opting for institutionalised networks or recruitment agencies to go abroad, migrants often rely on recommendations when choosing them. In spite of these recent developments, Bahna (2012), finds that social networks of compatriots who are already living abroad still entice CEE citizens to migrate, find a job and settle (e.g. Ryan et al., 2008). Therefore, the reliance on such networks has altered in the sense that CEE migrants act more independently and also consult professional agencies.

Forms of migration

As another aspect, also the forms of migration have changed and diversified and again reveal the variations within the group. Hence, apart from one-way migration, CEE post-accession migrants also choose circular forms of migration based on the intention they have for their stay. In this respect, Trevena (2013) distinguishes recent EU-8 migrants in the UK into three different types based on in-depth interviews with Polish university graduates in London. She speaks of "drifters" who come for post-materialist ends such as gaining experiences, learning the language, and travelling. While the drifters only stay on a temporary basis, the "career seekers" aiming at career advancement stay long-term. The third type, the "target earners", comes on a temporary basis to quickly earn a big amount of money to then invest in their home country upon their return. Accordingly, while "drifters" and "target earners" take up any employment that is flexible and pays well in the low-skilled sector, "career seekers" find themselves a position that promises the gain of new qualifications and upward mobility (ibid., p. 181). Building on the conceptualisation of different types of employment, Parutis (2014) conceives migration as a process. In her study on young Lithuanian and Polish migrants in the UK, she pointed out that these can also be thought of as phases that individual migrants pass through in the course of their stay based on their future orientations. Those aiming to settle down in the UK take up low-end jobs upon arrival in order to have an income and gain a foothold. After having become more familiar with the language and the new environment, they move on to a "better job" further investing in their human capital, and later on transition to their "dream job." This shows that migrants' aspirations change over time and that in-depth investigation is needed to capture these variations and developments.

However, not all migrants manage the transition from one phase to another. As Nowicka (2012) outlines, some migrants become trapped in migration. She criticises that Trevena (2013) includes explanatory factors at a micro, meso, and macro level for her analysis, but in the end gives most weight to the individuals' motivations when forming the types of migrants named above as well as the lack of an undertaken linkage of the three levels. Drawing on interviews with post-accession Polish migrants in the UK herself, Nowicka (2012) opens up a transnational social space including four stages of migration, namely one prior to leaving, one setting out, one of getting established, and the last one of an undefined future. From the first phase on, migrants link their own interests and motivations with macro level structural aspects such as the educational system, the labour market situation, or perceived job chances in both Poland and the UK as their country of destination. On a meso level, social networks consisting of friends who might already be abroad play an additional crucial role impacting their decision to migrate, as well as their readiness to take up employment under their level of skills. Under constant comparison of their situation in the UK with assumed possibilities in Poland as their country of origin, they remain in this transnational space in terms of the frame of reference towards which they are oriented. Not leaving the "Polish bubble" and staying in low-skilled jobs in the UK, they do not gain skills providing them with better job chances in the UK, or in Poland. Hence, they are trapped in these low-end jobs. This transnational perspective stresses the change from pre-accession, one-way migration patterns to diverse forms of mobility, and advocates the research of 'the human face' of migration to reveal these nuances.

Subjective perceptions of CEE migrants in the UK

Building thereon, Nowicka (2014) contributes to the discussion by drawing attention to the migrants' subjective perception of their situation, and to how they act based on that perception. With the help of narrative interviews with Polish migrants in the UK, she investigates narratives which the interviewees use to talk about the success or failure of their work-life in the UK. The interviewees were eager to construct their migration as success, thereby referring less to structural indicators such as their job placement, but drawing on their two-part reference frame mentioned above, namely the Polish as well as the UK context. With the help of this transnational orientation they weigh up their decision of whether to stay or to return. As Galasińska and Kozłowska (2009) find, this decision is significantly influenced by the migrants' assessment of a 'normal life'. Based on in-depth interviews and entries in relevant internet forums, they state that Polish migrants were primarily looking for 'normality' when leaving for the UK. 'Normality' from their point of view means having a job in which their earnings provide a certain level of security, and in which they receive respect from their superiors. Therefore, even if working under poor conditions and for little money compared to other UK residents, they themselves perceived their situation as an improvement from their situation in Poland. This comfort and ease which Polish migrants appreciated about their lives in the UK is also identified by Drinkwater and Garapich (2015) in a mixed-method approach. Particularly, with respect to welfare benefits on-site which they perceived as a safety net regarding their children's future, and which they would not have in Poland, they weighed up their options. Additionally, their experiences abroad together with met or unmet monetary expectations on-site determined the migrants' decision of whether to opt for settlement on-site or in their home country. Hence, again, the subjective evaluation of the migrant's individual situation in the context of broader institutional structures in two different countries of reference proves to give a better understanding of migration patterns than large-scale studies assessing structural indicators.

3.2 Institutional and cultural barriers to finding adequate employment and to induction at the work place

Persistent institutional barriers under liberal migration policies

A further point of criticism that Favell et al. (2007) raise, is the prevailing macro-economic notion that highly skilled migrants are welcomed by the host societies to fill market demands, and therefore do not encounter institutional barriers with respect to cultural or ideological constraints. This assumption is supported by the liberalisation of immigration policies for highly-skilled and the rhetoric of 'the race for the best minds' in many Western industrialised countries including Germany (see ch. 2.3). It further corresponds with the neo-liberal aim of the EU to become the "most competitive and dynamic knowledge-based economy in the world capable of sustainable economic growth with more and better jobs and greater social cohesion" ("Presidency Conlusions Council of the EU. Lisbon European Council. 23 and 24 March," 2000). This shall be achieved with the help of far reaching mobility rights enhancing the spatial as well as social mobility of EU citizens, supported by the harmonisations of academic and professional qualifications.

Cultural barriers to finding employment

Nevertheless, highly skilled migrants encounter difficulties that lie beyond the permission to work and that concern finding adequate employment. These barriers can be of a cultural and ideological nature and lead to the exclusion of highly skilled migrants from adequate employment. One example are different prevailing gender orders between the migrants' country of origin and the host country, as identified by Jungwirth (2008, 2011, 2012). Based on in-depth interviews with highly skilled female migrants from countries in the former SU in Germany, she found that they experienced a de-skilling by being recommended for un-skilled and gender-typical occupations on the part of the employment agency in Germany. All were trained and had gained work experience in STEM professions[11] in their countries of destination. While there it was common for women to work in such jobs, in (Western) Germany, technical professions have a strong male connotation. Hence, in spite of their high qualifications, these migrants were not regarded as adequate fit for practicing this profession in Germany by a governmental institution, although they had the legal right to work as engineers.

---

11   STEM refers to the academic disciplines of science, technology, engineering, and mathematics.

Institutional barriers to finding employment

Other immigrants in Germany experience institutional barriers that are based on their concrete professional qualifications. As Bauder (2005) found in interviews with employers, government bureaucrats, and NGO administrators in Berlin, *Aussiedler* who hold German citizenship (see ch. 2.1.1) and who were trained as engineers, teachers, or doctors in the former SU, faced de-skilling due to non-recognition in Germany. This was justified by the interviewees with the non-existence of certain professional and occupational titles in German, the lack of compatibility of the content learned for comparable and existing titles with the requirements in Germany, the different share of practical and theoretical parts during training, and the overall length thereof. In this respect, Bauder identifies ideological barriers with regard to the perception on the part of employers and government bureaucrats of the German training system as being superior to others, based on which this exclusion occurs.

Such circumstances apply particularly to highly skilled migrants trained in regulated professions in which the formal recognition of qualifications is administered by the respective professional association compared to non-regulated and more internationalised professions (Iredale, 2001). These considerations were empirically confirmed by Nohl (2010) who compared the job hunting process for migrant managers and migrant doctors in Canada and Germany based on narrative interviews with these migrants. While migrant managers had to prove their qualifications at the job, migrant physicians faced difficulties in obtaining the medical license necessary to practice on-site. The procedures to receive this license in Germany included tests of the applicants' state of knowledge run by the medical association. However, these tests were not transparent in terms of the tested knowledge to allow for adequate preparation. Hence, institutions in charge for the formal recognition of migrants' professional qualifications have a major impact on their adequate placement.

Institutional barriers to finding employment in the medical field

The medical profession is a prominent example for regulating the access to the profession with credentials (see also ch. 2.2.1). While to the best of my knowledge there are no empirical studies on the experiences of migrant doctors focusing on this specific aspect in Germany, there are respective studies thereon for EU countries in general and the Netherlands. Drawing on qualitative interviews with staff members of national health departments and university medical faculties, Herfs et al. (2007) state that the procedure migrant physicians from outside the European Economic Area (EEA)[12] have to undertake in order to acquire a license to practice, greatly varies across EU member

---

12   The EEA is a free trade area including all 28 European member countries, plus Iceland, Liechtenstein, and Norway.

states. In some countries, migrant doctors end up in unskilled jobs due to non-recognition of their qualifications. In others, the opportunity to catch up on the required qualifications is given for some cases. Nevertheless, non-EEA migrant doctors often do not stand the same chances to employment as local doctors do. This is illustrated for the case of the Netherlands by Huijskens et al. (2010). Based on in-depth interviews with non-EU migrant physicians, they find that their qualifications were not considered as equivalent, so that they had to complete subsequent training. Additionally, the physicians complained about a lack of information on the Dutch training and health care system, and a lack of financial support for the interim between receiving the medical license and looking for employment. Insufficient Dutch language skills are found to complicate employment possibilities.

Hence, even after having circumvented institutional barriers posed by governmental organisations and regulating bodies and having obtained the medical license, institutional barriers posed by potential employers are still in place. This underpins the claim made by Chapman and Iredale (1993) that formal acceptance of professional qualifications by the professional association is only one crucial step to take. For full recognition the informal acceptance by the employer must also be acquired. This is also the case for EU physicians. Although they are entitled to an automatic recognition of their credentials (see ch. 2.2.1), they are still likely to encounter institutional barriers beyond this formal recognition. However, as Bauder (2005) points out, the readiness to recognise foreign credentials and to employ migrant professionals additionally depends on the current labour market situation. While one of his interviewees argued that there was no need for medical doctors on-site at the time of the interview, these demands can change over time. Therefore, the question remains of how recognition processes take shape in times of labour shortages.

Workplace integration of highly skilled migrants

A further point of criticism raised by Favell et al. (2007) is that highly skilled migrants are not expected to encounter barriers such as discrimination or exploitation, or to struggle with glass ceilings in their jobs, and are not assumed to face challenges of induction at work. Therefore, research on highly skilled migrants primarily focuses on their job positioning rather than their integration in the workplace and accordingly, empirical research on this topic is scarce.

Nevertheless, the few existing empirical studies dealing with the occupational integration of migrants in their new work environments reveal that also highly-skilled encounter problems finding their way and are confronted with divergent workplace cultures, language barriers, and ethnic stereotyping. Mulholland and Ryan (2014) corroborate these problems in their study of French highly skilled migrants working in the finance sector in London. Their interviewees talked about the necessity for them to adapt to different ways of doing business, divergent styles of communicating and using language. Based on qualitative interviews with migrant women from Eastern European countries, Spain, and France working in technical professions in internationally operating companies located in Germany, Grigoleit (2012) shows that highly skilled migrants experienced barriers to integration at the new work place. Her interviewees were confronted with ethnic ascriptions based on national stereotypes. These were rather positive in the case of Western European, and rather negative in the case of Eastern European women, and were caused by the way the women dressed, as well as non-fluent German language skills. The migrant women did not receive professional or social recognition before mastering the German language – even if the company was internationally aligned and the working language was supposed to be English. Therefore, high human capital in terms of professional qualifications alone, do not guarantee smooth induction. Even in professions that are classified as highly internationalised (such as finance), country-specific expectations can hamper the transfer and the application of knowledge and skills.

Workplace integration of migrant physicians

As for highly skilled migrants in general, also in medical migration research corresponding studies on migrant physicians' experiences in the workplace are scarce. However, the existing ones come to similar findings. In spite of the formal recognition of their qualifications, some migrant doctors experience forms of de-skilling (being assigned to tasks that lie below their qualifications), or exclusion from specialized training opportunities (see Humphries et al. (2014) for their study of non-EU medical doctors in Irish hospitals). Jinks et al. (2000) find that differences in the training between the UK and the migrant doctors' respective home country, superiors were sceptical and did not trust migrants' credentials (see also: Tjadens, Eckert, & Weilandt, 2012, p. 25ff.). Difficulties with communication in the local language was frequently mentioned to be a massive barrier to practicing medicine abroad, particularly since the medical profession is very interactive (den Adel, Blauw, Dobson, Hoesch, & Salt, 2004).

In their study on migrant physicians in German hospitals, Ognyanova et al. (2014) find that migrant doctors perceived the German language as a major difficulty in finding their way in a German hospital. They stress that migrant physicians who had the chance to participate in a preparation class which was offered by private providers in Germany, greatly benefited thereof. These include not only language training, but also introductions into the German culture as well as the culture in German hospitals[13]. Since different cultural habits

13   Concerning such integration classes see Srur (2010).

and ways of interacting with patients and colleagues were frequently emphasised, the necessity of integration measures helping the migrant doctors to find their way in an unfamiliar working environment were also stressed elsewhere (Fellmer, 2008; Kopetsch, 2009). These findings emphasise the large impact that the attitude of patients and co-workers has in that situation and stresses the fact that recognition of professional qualifications is not only a formal, but also a social process continuing during the migrants' work routine on-site. Furthermore, they reveal the significance that is attributed to cultural and linguistic knowledge in this concrete professional context that according to the authors has to be supported with the help of induction measures.

Within the scope of the Work-Int project, an EU funded project that was conducted in five European cities, Kovacheva and Grewe (2015b) focus on the workplace integration of EU as well as non-EU migrant doctors and nurses in hospitals in the city of Hamburg. They conducted qualitative interviews with migrant doctors and nurses, hospital managers and representatives of work councils, as well as external stakeholders such as policy makers or representatives of professional associations and trade unions in 2014. In the employers' perspective, they find that the Hamburg hospitals did not experience a shortage of physicians. Therefore, they chose to employ migrant doctors for whom little bureaucratic effort was required, and who master the German language. Accordingly, most migrant doctors on-site had been living in Germany previously, and did not migrate for work explicitly, but had accompanied or joined their partner in Germany. On the part of the hospital, no measures to support the migrant doctors during their initial phase were taken, apart from help with bureaucratic procedures, occasional language classes and mentoring arrangements. The migrant doctors, however, often felt overwhelmed with the accompanying expectation to immediately know local codes of conduct and work routines. Again, particularly the language posed a barrier, but also differing work cultures. While these occasionally lead to mistrust and disrespect on the part of nurses and patients, the respondents received support from their colleagues in getting used to the local standards. Particularly, a mentoring programme was appreciated that due to a good staff situation allowed mentor and mentee extra time during the daily routine. However, since these hospitals in Hamburg benefited from a generous staffing, the question remains in how far small, rural facilities are able to provide migrant physicians with according circumstances, and whether they find different means to support migrant doctors in their hospitals.

Wolanik Boström and Öhlander (2012)[14], however, detect very subtle differences between the migrant physicians' and the local work cultures to be crucial that would not necessarily be ruled out with the help of induction

---

14 See also Wolanik Boström and Öhlander (2011).

measures. They present a very dense and illustrative study on the topic of migrant physicians' integration at the workplace based on ethnographic research on Polish migrant doctors in Swedish hospitals. They find accordingly, the migrant physicians perceived an initial mistrust in their competencies and had to perform basic, unfavourable tasks. Additionally, their de-skilling was expressed in lower salaries compared to those of native physicians. The migrant doctors found themselves to be beginners again, not being able to apply their skills the ways they used to, due to differing cultural traits[15] and language problems. Language and the way of expressing oneself proved to be crucial, not just with respect to communicating with patients, but also with colleagues, and superiors. Especially elderly professors treated 'fine' Swedish as crucial indicator for competence and trustworthiness. At the same time, more informal situations posed a challenge to the migrant physicians. This was based on a different degree of formality and thus expressing oneself that the Polish physicians first had to learn. However, the degree of professionalism was not only assessed based on language, but also based on the way of dressing oneself. Used to a more formal dress code in Polish hospitals, and a different perception of appropriate clothing, – in particular for women – Polish migrant physicians were viewed with suspicion. Especially female Polish physicians came into conflicts with female care personnel during the first phase of their work abroad. Apart from differing cultural traits and the given language difficulties further reasons for the Polish physicians' experiences could be negative stereotypes of Eastern Europeans prevalent in Sweden. Hence, local professional norms and values hamper the professional integration of migrant physicians still after having found employment.

Physicians' professional identity after migration

Focussing on the aspect of professional identity, Shuval (2000) and Bernstein (2000) deal with the question of how issues of downgrading and a related loss of status after migration impact the migrant physicians' self-perception. They base their research on the case of medical doctors from the former SU immigrating to Canada, the US, and Israel in 1990. The data was collected using narrative interviews about the physicians' life stories in 1991, which were completed and followed up with surveys via mail in 1991, 1993 and 1995. Shuval (2000) emphasises the salience the professional role has to physicians and the high degree of professional identity. She finds that they were determined to urgently restore the status they had held before migration as its loss through down-grading being employed in rather unfavourable specialisations and positions in their host countries, posed a threat to their professional identity. In the same vein, Bernstein (2000) identifies the perception of the own

---

15 Very illustrative in this respect is the auto-ethnographic study by Harris (2011) on bodily adjustment of migrant physicians in an overseas hospital environment.

skills as being equal to the ones of native physicians, as well as recognition on the part of colleagues and patients as crucial for the migrant doctor's well-being in Israel. Hence, not only the formal, but also informal recognition are crucial for a perceived integration and thus the well-being of migrant physicians on-site. Relatedly, again the subjective perception of the migrant's situation gives a deeper insight into the success of migration than the surveying of structural job placement.

Drawing on the work of Bernstein (2000) and Shuval (2000), Ribeiro (2008) finds that the formal recognition of professional qualifications is only one dimension of the successful integration of migrant physicians, and points to the social, cultural, political, and symbolic dimensions of this process impacting the individual's professional identity. In her qualitative study on migrant physicians and care personnel from Spain, Moldova, Russia, and the Ukraine in the Portuguese health care system, she researched their occupational integration based on biographical interviews. Her findings reveal that in spite of the formal recognition of qualifications respondents were excluded from further training or certain responsibilities. Furthermore, the differing cultural contexts, the health workers stem from and were trained and socialised in, posed great challenges to their successful integration in terms of differing codes of conduct. Care personnel and medical doctors encountered language difficulties, discrimination, and conflicts with native colleagues. Thus, she concludes that national arrangements of the health care systems and the salience of cultural contexts remain also in times of globalisation and European integration, and that market interests proved to be stronger than shared professional identities.

To conclude, even after having found employment highly skilled migrants encounter various difficulties challenging their induction at the work place. These difficulties range from language issues, a social and cultural disjuncture with their ethnic origin, and the workplace culture. Disturbances based on subtle differences with regard to codes of conduct, dress codes and use of language reflect mechanisms of closure exerted by the professional associations. Nonetheless, there is only little empirical data on integration problems faced by migrant doctors.

3.3 Conceptual approaches to the transfer of skills

Breaking up the human capital approach

The third point of criticism Favell et al. (2007) raise, is the postulation of a human capital perspective that without further ado highly skilled migrants can transfer their professional knowledge and skills from one national context to another. Human capital theorists act on the assumption of rational actors and rational organisations operating according to market rule, striving for the highest gain possible. Regarding migration, human capital theory assumes a free market in which migrants can find work under the conditions of fair competition, based on their professional qualifications and competences. It is in the interest of the respective employer to hire migrant workers and professionals according to their level of skills. If this venture fails and migrants experience a mismatch of qualifications and forms of de-skilling, human capital theory identifies the reason for that in a lack of information about the respective qualifications on the part of the employer (Becker, 1993).

However, the empirical studies referenced above (ch. 3.2) show that human capital, (i.e. professional qualifications and skills), do not have a fixed value as suggested in the human capital approach. In order to emphasise this relativity, Csedő (2008) draws attention to professional skills as social constructs stating that professional qualifications that are regarded as valuable in one context, are not necessarily regarded as such in another. Accordingly, she distinguishes between *highly qualified* migrants on the one and *highly skilled* migrants on the other hand. While the former possess qualifications that are generally regarded as high, the latter possess qualifications that are regarded as high in a particular work context and therefore applicable therein. Whether or not this applies is the result of a social process in which the highly qualified migrant negotiates the value of their skills with the potential employer. It thus depends on the capability of the migrant to signal the value of their credentials as well as on the perception and assessment thereof by the employer.

Institutional approach to skill transfer

Depicted above (ch. 3.2), regulated professions such as medicine upstream to negotiations with the employer via professional associations. In this context, not only social, but also cultural implications play a major role to skill recognition. In order to understand this process, some scholars draw on an institutional approach (e.g. Allsop et al., 2009; Salaff & Greve, 2003). This perspective focuses on the influence of institutional interests on the part of the state, markets, and professional associations (Fligstein, 2001). With regard to the professions, Salaff and Greve (2003) argue that a sequence of career steps starting with an apprenticeship and followed by career steps bound to the takeover of tasks with increasing responsibilities has been established creating a certain path dependency. Hence, certain career achievements are expected which serve to signal competence. However, these achievements are not universal, but embedded in social structures including certain patterns of behaviour and norms (Granovetter, 1985) and are based "on a shared conception of the problems to be solved and the approaches to be employed, and, indeed, what constitutes a 'solution'" (ibid. Scott, 2008, p. 225, original emphasis). Due to the large power of many professional associations, these shared values translate into set standards and thus become institutionalised in the structure of the labour market in the form of a professional order or professional culture.

Professions, then, can be understood as being cultures similar to organizational cultures in so far as they exist within an historical context and professional environment, which, together with the societal culture, shape their operating practices and professional codes, beliefs, values, and ceremonies (Bloor & Dawson, 1994, p. 283)

Hence, internal markets are created that exclude those who are not regarded as matching the established standards on-site. However, while this approach manages to explain institutional barriers to accreditation, it falls short on explaining more subtle mechanisms of skill devaluation that lie beyond institutionalised standards.

Cultural capital approach to skill transfer

A different approach to explain the accreditation process run by professional associations is the adoption of the notion of 'cultural capital' put forward by the French sociologist Pierre Bourdieu. For instance, Bauder (2003) conceives the non-recognition of immigrants' qualifications on the part of professional associations as intentional. Drawing on Bourdieu, he stresses its systemic character by conceptualising the credentials migrants bring as *institutionalised cultural capital* referring to Bourdieu's understanding of social reproduction taking place in educational systems. In the same way as educational systems define standards according to middle-class cultural modes, professional associations define the entry requirements to their profession in a cultural mode matching their own standards. Thus, they exclude immigrants who gained their cultural capital elsewhere and therefore adhere to different cultural modes.

In a later publication on the assessment of engineers' professional qualifications by the respective professional body in Canada, Girard and Bauder (2007) identify the requirement of local work experience as a less formalised form of capital, which they refer to as 'habitus'. With 'habitus' Bourdieu describes schemes of perception, that are shared within social groups organising their behaviour. The authors employ this notion to capture the more subtle rules guiding professional associations' expectations of behaviour. These expectations are oriented towards codes of conduct, such as representation skills, norms of workplace behaviour, or a dress code, which are established on-site and additionally underlie criteria such as age, gender, or ethnic origin. Again, those not falling into the defined categories are excluded. Thus, the professional associations aim to protect their own position by giving preference to 'domestic' members and denying formal recognition of immigrants' qualifications due to both their institutionalised cultural capital, i.e. their credentials as well as their habitus based on their membership in certain social groups.

Hence, the authors manage to capture less standardised aspects leading to a devaluation of professional skills that are linked to the professional context. While they remain on the level of accreditation, the concepts could also be taken to the level of workplace integration explaining irritations that might occur based on deviations from locally established professional routines and standards. Nevertheless, in the way they are employed by Bauder (2003) and Girard and Bauder (2007), these concepts are limited to professional aspects not able to cover aspects that lie beyond this professional sphere. In this respect, Nohl et al. (2014, 2010b) have gone further. Apart from the social and cultural processes of the recognition of immigrants' qualifications, they further emphasise the symbolic process of skill recognition in terms of a devaluation of cultural capital due to the holders' ethnic origin, which also Girard and Bauder (2007) alluded to. Nohl et al. (2010) argue that even if migrants' institutionalised cultural capital is formally recognised, migrants can still experience a symbolic devaluation thereof at the work place. This symbolic devaluation of the migrants' cultural capital can be based on their migrant status, their status as newcomers, or a poor account of the local language. Hence, "[t]he value of cultural capital is reduced indirectly as a result of suspicion of 'the other'" (Nohl et al., 2014, p. 157, original emphasis). In this case, symbolic struggles take place in which the value of the migrants' cultural capital is negotiated and can also be valorised when trust can be established. However, symbolic exclusion can also persist and find expression, for instance, in the exclusion from certain tasks, or the permanent assignment to tasks, e.g. if a Polish doctor's responsibility in a German hospital would be limited to taking care of Polish patients.

Thus, in the application of Nohl et al. (2014; 2010b), the cultural capital approach is able to capture mechanism of symbolic devaluation complementing its application by Bauder (2003) and Girard and Bauder (2007), which is focused on the social and cultural assessment of qualifications by professional associations. Thus, they cover subtle mechanisms that the institutional approach cannot depict in such a systematic way. However, the institutional approach is helpful for understanding the significance of professional standards for the respective institution. Hence, all of these approaches are valuable for understanding the process of skill assessment – it's social, cultural, and symbolic implications – and inform the present study.

3.4 Identified research gaps and the contribution of this study

In the following, I summarise the main points made in the literature review with respect to the dichotomisation of groups of migrants, the exploration of newly emerging migration patterns, the disregard of cultural and institutional barriers that highly skilled migrants might encounter in finding adequate employment as well as in integrating at the work place, and conceptual approaches to the transfer of qualifications and skills. I stress the identified research gaps, and the work I build on by investigating the recent migration of CEE physicians to Germany.

First, in spite of their status as EU citizens, the perception of CEE migrants as free movers and thus equal EU citizens has failed to appear. With regard to the German context, CEE migrants are discussed in the same manner as prior to EU accession, namely, as low skilled migrants in low-end, gender-typical jobs. With regard to post-accession East-West migration to the UK, this polarisation has dissolved at least insofar that they are visible as highly skilled migrants. However, this is reduced to their educational background and does not apply to their job placement abroad. Accordingly, CEE post-accession migrants are hardly visible in their capacity as EU movers, and are not perceived as such, for instance, on the part of employers. Hence, I aim to close this research gap and contribute to the visibility of CEE highly skilled migrants – both men and women – in the upper sector of the German and hence, Western European labour markets. I wish to counteract the one-sided perception of CEE migrants as economically driven and placed in low-end jobs by investigating the intra-EU migration of CEE physicians as 'middling migrants' and thus, as 'regular' EU movers.

Second, the hitherto dichotomisation between 'low skilled' and 'highly skilled' is further softened in research on post-accession migration from CEE countries to the UK. Acknowledging the fact, that also highly skilled migrants can encounter barriers to adequate employment, scholars explore variations in migration patterns encompassing migration motives, strategies, and forms that are employed by CEE migrants. Empirical evidence shows that there is an individualisation and diversification of migration patterns. Since changing patterns in recent East-West migration have not been studied in-depth in Germany, I contribute to the body of research on East-West post-accession migration with the depiction of the case of CEE physicians in German hospitals.

Third, contrary to the assumption that highly skilled migrants do not encounter cultural and institutional barriers to finding employment matching their skills as well as to integrate in the new working environment, particularly qualitative, in-depth studies have shown otherwise. Especially migrants in regulated professions, such as the medical one, struggle to obtain the formal recognition by the respective professional associations. The recognition procedures underlie cultural and ideological patterns excluding those who gained their qualifications abroad. Similar processes are in place with respect to the rarely studied workplace integration of highly skilled migrants in general, and migrant physicians in particular. The few existing studies refer to discrimination and exclusion based on language proficiency, ethnic origin, and differing work cultures including subtle aspects such as ways of expressing oneself, codes of conduct, or a certain dress code. For the case of migrant physicians, research reveals that symbolic exclusion based on such aspects, just as experienced forms of deskilling, pose a threat to their professional identity and thus, their self-esteem. In conclusion, apart from formal recognition, also informal recognition plays a crucial role for the success of a migrant's labour market integration, and can hence be conceived as limitation to mobility. Since this issue is hardly researched with regard to highly-skilled, I aim to contribute to the state of research by adding further empirical data in this respect. Thus, I emphasise the significance of both formal and informal recognition for the (self-perceived) positioning of migrants. Moreover, I address the open question of how these cultural and institutional barriers alter under the condition of pressing labour market shortages.

Fourth, while the empirical evidence presented above renders the economic perspective suggested by the human capital approach obsolete, other conceptual approaches manage to capture the variety of factors that impact the process of skill recognition and transfer. The institutional perspective helps to understand institutional mechanism of exclusion through non-recognition and the ideological as well as political impact thereon. Approaches employing Bourdieu's notion of cultural capital and habitus complete this perspective by stressing crucial subtle aspects ingrained in professional socialisation, but also symbolic processes of exclusion that refer to the migrants' status as foreigner. While these approaches help to understand the mechanisms of skill devaluation as well as valorisation, and thus explain the objective positioning of immigrants, I aim to focus on the migrants' subjective perception thereof which has hardly been studied before, but in these few studies has proven to provide a valuable insight into their action orientation. Therewith, I contribute to the account of research on skill recognition by not only stating and explaining potential devaluations, but by exploring its 'human face' through investigating the meaning thereof for the migrants.

3.5 Research questions

Immigration policies for CEE citizens to Germany were vastly liberalised in the course of the EU accession of their countries (see ch. 2.1.2). Moreover, the access for migrant physicians to practice medicine in Germany was tremendously facilitated in response to the increasing demand for medical doctors. On paper, the transfer of the CEE migrant physicians' qualifications appears uncomplicated; their credentials are formally recognised, and the physicians should be deemed equal to native physicians. Despite this, research reveals at least three critical barriers that might impede the smooth transfer of the CEE migrant physicians' professional knowledge and skills to the German hospitals.

Firstly, despite the automatic formal recognition of EU physicians' professional qualifications resulting from the EU directive on the harmonisation of professional qualifications, the medical associations at Laender level make the final decision about the recognition. Therefore, proof of proficiency in the local language, or familiarity with locally established professional standards weighs heavily upon the decision to recognize medical credentials. Professional associations endeavour to maintain their prerogative of interpretation via these mechanisms of closure, while the local hospital administrations decide whether or not to employ migrant physicians. Both the readiness to recognise foreign credentials and to employ migrant physicians, depends on the current staff situation (Bauder, 2005; Girard & Bauder, 2007). These findings imply that the facilitated access to the German medical license is a necessary, but not sufficient condition for the adequate positioning of CEE migrant doctors at the German labour market.

Secondly, symbolic devaluation of the migrant physicians' professional status in their new working environment is a common phenomenon, as the literature on the recognition of cultural capital of highly skilled migrants by Nohl et al. (2014; 2010b) suggests. Symbolic devaluation occurs when the migrants' professional qualifications do not receive informal recognition, which can be the case in spite of their formal recognition (Nohl, Ofner, et al., 2010). This can be expressed through discrimination and symbolic exclusion based, for instance, on national stereotypes or deficits in the local language (Grigoleit, 2012).

Finally, although professional qualifications in terms of credentials are harmonised across the EU, this does not apply to implicit professional codes of conduct and cultural modes. These diverge between different countries based on the socialisation in different medical systems (Ribeiro, 2008; Wolanik Boström & Öhlander, 2012). Therefore, differing work cultures and routines could impede the induction at the workplace in spite of the formal recognition of professional qualifications and adequate experience.

Given these remaining barriers that pertain to the situation of CEE migrant physicians in German hospitals, my concern is that irrespective of the liberalisations at policy level, the induction and incorporation of the migrant doctors at the actual workplace is insufficient. The shortage of physicians might be decreased by the recruitment of migrant doctors, however, there is a serious risk that this work force is not supported and valued appropriately, nor effectively utilised. Formal recognition of qualifications is just one component in sustainably addressing staff shortages. Another critical component is to provide migrants with a supportive and acknowledging environment in order to ensure their equal participation in the labour market. Related dissatisfaction on the part of the migrant physicians and the potential wish of return migration or re-migration to another country could imply that the efforts undertaken by the German government, the medical association, and the hospital administrations to meet the shortage of physicians are unsustainable.

Therefore, I explore the circumstances under which the migration of CEE migrant physicians to German hospitals occurs, and how this process is perceived by the migrant doctors. Thus, I aim to investigate the remaining limits of mobility against the backdrop of the liberalisation of immigration policies and access regulations. To this end, I propose the following general research question, which is broken down into three subordinate research questions:

How do the migration of CEE physicians and their recruitment in German hospitals take place under the conditions of liberalised immigration policies to Germany and facilitated access authorisations to the medical profession?

I.   How is this form of East-West migration characterised in terms of
   a.   how the recruitment and induction of CEE migrant physicians is organised on the part of the hospital administrations?
   b.   the motivations and strategies of the CEE physicians to migrate in order to practice medicine in German hospitals?
II. How do the CEE migrant physicians perceive their situation, and what are their coping mechanisms based on this perception?

The first subordinate research question is meant to capture the nature of this medical East-West migration including both the perspective of employers and migrant physicians. Research question I, dimensions *a*, targets the employers' perspective in the organisation of the recruitment process of CEE migrant physicians on behalf of the hospital administrations. Given the current shortage of medical doctors, I am interested in recruitment strategies in general and specific measures taken to induct the migrant doctors on-site. By including the employers' perspective, I describe the institutional context the migrant doctors encounter on-site. Thus, I aim to comprehensively explore the underlying patterns of this medical migration to Germany in terms of a new form of post-accession East-West migration. Question I, dimension *b* focuses on the migrant doctors' perspective. It addresses migration motives and the strategies of migration employed by the CEE physicians under study. Thus, the first subordinate research question is meant to explore the nature of this medical migration to Germany, including its circumstances, as well as the expectations the migrants attach to it.

The second subordinate research question addresses the migrant doctors' evaluation of their overall situation, including a retrospective evaluation of their original migration choice and prospective future plans. By taking this biographical perspective I assess how migrant doctors perceive their situation in German hospitals against the backdrop of the experiences they have on-site, how they cope with it, and ultimately, how their experiences impact their biographical orientations in terms of their inclination to stay in Germany. For instance, initial expectations towards migrating to Germany could alter the migrant physicians' original plans to stay or leave (see also Breckner, 2007, p. 118). To this end, I draw on the theoretical concept of *biographical uncertainty* (e.g. Bonß & Zinn, 2005; Reiter, 2010; Zinn, 2004).

The concept of biographical uncertainty is based on the assumption that in the course of modernisation and corresponding individualisation, the world has become increasingly uncertain in many respects (Beck, 1992). One aspect is the erosion of the formerly "institutionalised life course" (Kohli, 2007), the reliable sequence of life course stages, such as training, paid employment, household formation, and retirement. With the change of long established norms and structures – the foundation of the institutionalised life course – biographical certainty dissolved. On the one hand, this led to more and different life-stage possibilities. On the other hand, individuals were also forced to actively plan their life (Bonß & Zinn, 2005). This individual life planning entails the pressure to make the right life choices. Since the outcome of made decisions is difficult to predict and can thus be unexpected, the individualisation in respect to one's life course results in biographical uncertainty (Zinn, 2004). Biographical uncertainty can, thus, be understood as the disability to anticipate the contingency of upcoming events in the life course and to react to their realisation (Bonß & Zinn, 2005, p. 187).

International migration, i.e. the transition from one national context to another, is one example causing biographical uncertainty, since transitions "(…) are characterized by an inherent uncertainty concerning outcome and consequences for the future" (Reiter, 2010). In the case of migration, this pertains since norms and values that shape expectations differ between countries; for instance, with regard to the notion of a *normal* life course (Bonß & Zinn, 2005; Nowicka, 2014, p. 74). Finding adequate employment abroad is further complicated, for instance, due to a different official language, as well as unknown expectations and professional standards held by employers (Nohl et al., 2014). Accordingly, migrants experience uncertainty in terms of what to expect after migration, and in terms of the fear to fail in meeting own expectations and visions. Junge (2014) conceives the notion of failure as a crucial condition for action. Individuals take action in order to address or prevent failure. Thus, he locates the notion of failure in action theory. However, since "(…) failure is relative to a normatively fixed, locally and historically produced, expectation of success (…)" (Nowicka, 2014, p. 75), the notion of failure as well as ways of coping with failure must be assessed in context (Junge, 2014). Consequently, this approach allows analysing social values and norms guiding the perception and coping strategies of migrant physicians in German hospitals.

Zinn (2004) identifies two different kinds of coping strategies that are employed in order to address uncertainty and thus the risk to fail, namely *certainty constructions* and *protective actions*. The former "refer to expectations, that is, the level of interpretations" (ibid. 203). Being confronted with uncertainty, the individual reinterprets the situation in order to restore certainty. The latter refers to action strategies that are targeted at "achieving certainty in the sense of protection against events that are assessed to be negative" (ibid.). Through research questions *I* and *II*, I investigate the circumstances under which the post-accession migration of CEE migrant doctors to German hospitals takes place, which barriers they encounter, and how their experience onsite impacts their evaluation of their current and prospective work-life situation. Thus, I shed light on the question of which factors are decisive for the job satisfaction, and thus the sustainable incorporation of migrant physicians in Germany.

4 Research Design and Methods

After presenting the state of research as well as the research questions of the study, this chapter depicts the underlying research design and the methods employed. The chapter starts out by defining the research interest and the approach taken to research the phenomenon under scrutiny (4.1). It then outlines the methods used for data collection (4.2), and the sampling procedure, as well as the final case selection (4.3). The chapter continues with the description of the data analysis (4.4) and finishes with the discussion of methodical limitations of the study (4.5).

4.1 Research interest and analytic approach

In order to answer the above stated research questions (ch. 3.5), I employ a qualitative-exploratory research design in the interpretative paradigm, reconstructing collectively shared, as well as subjective, interpretation patterns of crucial actors involved in the phenomenon under study (Rubin & Rubin, 2012, p. 19f.). The exploratory approach is applied due to the novelty of the migration and recruitment process of CEE migrant doctors to German hospitals, and the lack of studies focusing thereon, as previously elaborated on (ch. 3).

The research interest is two-fold in its empirical application. I am interested in how the above stated bureaucratic facilitations and the demand for physicians is reflected in institutional terms at the hospital level. Therefore, I investigate the practices and perceptions of the hospital administrations in their endeavour to recruit and induct the CEE migrant physicians. The gained findings serve as a complementary source of information (Bogner, Littig, & Menz, 2014, p. 23) forming the institutional context of the recruitment and professional integration of migrant doctors. Therefore, I am interested in *procedural knowledge* from the employers' side (ibid., p. 18) which includes knowledge about, and experience with recruitment strategies (1), supportive measures to assist the migrant physicians with the obtainment of the medical license (2), as well as with their professional induction in the hospital (3). Informing about a procedure from a certain point of view, *procedural knowledge* resembles practical knowledge, and is bound to an individual carrying interpretative knowledge at the same time (ibid.). Hence, it additionally reveals the attitudes and stances guiding the action and decision-making of the person in charge. However, I am not interested in the respondents' personal or individual interpretations, but in collectively shared interpretations as representatives of this special group (Helfferich, 2011, p. 33), i.e. in their capacity as representatives of the hospital administrations. Since this kind of knowledge is bound to the individual, it could not be gained by other means of data collection.

Apart from the employers' depiction of the situation under study, I am interested in the migrant physicians' migration motivations and strategies, as well as their experiences vis-á-vis this institutional context, and the way they respond to them. Therefore, I focus on their subjective perception of the conditions the migrant physicians encounter in the German hospitals, and the coping strategies they develop based thereon. I draw on "biographical action research" (Zinn, 2010) which focuses on the way individuals deal with specific problems in a certain situation. Hence, this approach is not concerned with explanations based on an individual's life course or biographical identity. "The significant question of this kind of research is how different action logics or interpretation patterns come together or are linked to specific contexts, rather than to the personality" (ibid.). Accordingly, in order to capture these contexts, I concentrate on the references the migrant doctors make when articulating their individual interpretation patterns, and their action logics. Drawing on Nowicka (2014), I therefore pay attention to references in terms of who or what is seen as causing uncertainty or the notion of failure, from which perspective circumstances are evaluated as successes or failures, and the time frame in which the migrant doctors set their aims and expectations (ibid., p. 77). Thus, I aim to understand the relevance structures of the migrant doctors for the evaluation of their overall situation.

Both the employers' and the migrant physicians' perspectives are understood as complementary, together providing an encompassing understanding of the migration and recruitment process. In the presentation of the findings, I first depict the employers' perspective (ch. 5) in order to set the institutional context of the study, followed by the depiction of the migrant physicians' perspective (ch. 6). The findings of the former are discussed individually in the interim conclusions of the respective chapter and integrated in the chapter of the physicians' perspective where connecting points arise. I link the findings to both subordinate research questions in the final conclusions in order to address the general research question. The methods applied in the two different empirical inquiries are presented following the same order as the depiction of the respective findings.

4.2 Data collection

4.2.1 Expert interviews

Method of data collection

Many different actors on various levels such as state, medical association, as well as hospital administrations and staff, and not least patients, shape the context of the recruitment and incorporation of migrant physicians. This entails a process that is ridden with prerequisites. Since I am interested in the physicians' integration at the work place, I focus on the hospital level, and particularly, on the recruitment procedure and the provision of incorporation measures on the part of the hospital administration. Therefore, I conducted expert interviews with HR managers and medical directors. They were chosen since they are in charge for the employment of medical doctors in the hospitals. While HR managers are responsible for HR issues in a hospital in general, medical directors are physicians who are consulted for the employment of medical doctors as one aspect of their responsibilities. Medical directors in large hospitals are often employed full-time, whereas in smaller facilities they are recruited from the group of head physicians and hold this office extra-professionally. In any case, due to their capacity of being medical doctors themselves, I intended to gain an internal professional and medical perspective on the recruitment and incorporation process, complementing the more economically oriented one of the HR managers. Thus, I aim to capture two relevant orientations represented by the hospital administrations.

Hence, both HR managers and medical directors are crucial actors, having specialised knowledge on the recruitment and incorporation of migrant physicians in their facilities at their disposal (Przyborski & Wohlrab-Sahr, 2009, p. 131). Additionally, they significantly impact and effect the situation under study due to their decision-making authority (Bogner et al., 2014, p. 13; Meuser & Nagel, 2009, p. 43ff.). They actively shape and determine the circumstances the migrant doctors encounter on-site as well as the migrant doctors' scope for action. Hence, understanding the HR managers' and medical directors' action logic will help to better comprehend the institutional context the migrant doctors' encounter at German hospitals.

Interview guide

The expert interviews were conceptualised as semi-structured interviews (Przyborski & Wohlrab-Sahr, 2009, p. 138; Rubin & Rubin, 2012, p. 31) based on an interview guide that consisted of six thematic sections, namely, reasons for the recruitment of migrant physicians (I), strategies of attracting and incorporating migrant physicians (II), interactions between migrant physicians on the one hand, and medical colleagues, other hospital staff, and patients on the other (III), applied general human resource strategies (IV), perspective reflections on the shortage of medical doctors and its development in Germany in general (V), and reflections, evaluations, and future estimations with regard to the employment of migrant physicians in one's own facility in particular (VI) (for the full interview guide, see attachment i).

Interview questions gathered in interview guides can be developed based on general knowledge as well as existing literature and preliminary research (Rubin & Rubin, 2012, p. 134f.). For this study I drew on both everyday knowledge and preparatory readings on the topic under scrutiny, and broader related subjects such as labour migration, the medical profession, and hospital procedures. All of the interviews started by inviting the experts to introduce themselves in their position in order to acknowledge the interviewees' status as experts (Przyborski & Wohlrab-Sahr, 2009, p. 135) and to provide a smooth opener giving the interviewees the opportunity to get used to the interview situation (ibid., p. 80). Apart from knowledge questions concerning the process of recruitment and incorporation targeted mainly at gaining information on the procedure undertaken, further questions focused on experiences with certain strategies and measures, and asked for evaluation and reflection. These latter questions were used to encourage conscious reasoning and thus attain the interviewees' interpretative patterns and attached meanings (Helfferich, 2011, p. 106). With the help of a final question asking the respondents' whether they wanted to add anything, the setting of own relevance structures was further ensured (Patton, 2002, p. 379). The course of the thematic sections and related interview questions followed the chronological order of the recruitment process in order to facilitate the narrative thread. However, as common for qualitative interviews, in the actual interview situation the guide was handled with flexibility responding openly to the interviewees' relevance structures (ibid., p. 181).

Course of the interview

The experts were generally very open to participating in the interviews and showed interest in the topic which led to informative and insightful interviews that allowed me to retrieve the desired information. Yet, it appeared that the interview questions regarding the reasons and strategies for recruiting physicians from abroad seemed more plausible and intuitive for HR managers and medical directors representing rural hospitals, rather than those representing city hospitals who replied to these questions in a somewhat cumbersome way. This might be due to the former having had to engage with this procedure for a much longer period, whereas the latter often did not engage in active recruitment. However, one respondent in particular from a city hospital was eager to present the situation in his hospital as unproblematic in terms of filling vacancies. In the beginning of the interview he stated that only one or two CEE migrant physicians would be employed in the hospital. In the course of the interview he then recalled more and more, and in the end of interview he concluded that maybe he should start thinking about how to address the issue of recruiting and incorporating migrant physicians in a better way. Reasons for this behaviour could be that he felt being dependent on migrant physicians taints the reputation of the hospital, or that indeed he did not regard occasional shortages as a general problem. In any case, the interview seems to have raised his awareness for the subject.

One of the medical directors of a rural hospital with many CEE migrant physicians was very eager to present their presence in the hospital as unproblematic. The way in which he repeatedly stressed this good rapport, however, seemed dubious. Again, he was keen to present the facility in a favourable way, which could reveal either ignorance or unawareness on his part, since I know from the interviews with migrant physicians on-site that the situation is not as uncomplicated as depicted by the medical director. Another respondent of a rural hospital with a number of CEE migrant physicians was very cautious in the way he expressed himself making an effort to use politically correct language when talking about the situation under scrutiny. Like almost all of the other interviewees, he stressed the cultural enrichment that the migrant physicians brought to the hospital when being asked to reflect upon the situation in the end of the interview. Particularly in this case, this statement appeared to be a matter of social desirability rather than a genuine sentiment.

The questions targeted at the cooperation between migrant doctors on the one hand, and German (-trained) physicians as well as other hospital staff on the other hand, could not be answered in detail by the HR managers since they are not present at ward during the daily routine. Here, the responses of those medical directors who were practicing at the same time were more helpful. Questions regarding general human resource strategies, for instance, in terms of how to deal with extra hours or measures to address the issue of compatibility of job and family in the case of physicians were only posed to HR managers. However, these turned out to be not employable for the research interest, since the migrant physicians did not relate to these issues. While the HR managers, for instance, elaborated on measures for physicians on paternal leave to remain in touch with the hospital, this topic was not relevant to the migrant physicians at the time of the interview.

The expert interviews were conducted in the experts' offices, and lasted between 20 and 88 minutes with an average time of 43 minutes. Before starting the interview, the respondents were informed about the broad research interest and the procedure. They were asked to sign a form giving their consent to the recording of the interview and the use of the gained material. Altogether nine expert interviews were conducted between November 2012 and March 2013.

4.2.2 Problem-centred interviews

Method of data collection

Problem-centred interviews (PCI) (Witzel & Reiter, 2012) were conducted with CEE migrant physicians. This form of interviewing was developed by Witzel. The term "problem-centred" refers to a relevant problem that is conceived by the researcher in the form of flexibly handled prior knowledge on the one hand. On the other hand it refers to the subjective understanding of this problem on the part of the interviewee (Witzel, 1982, p. 69). The prior knowledge the researcher has inevitably acquired in preparing the subject of the study is inductively complemented with the interviewees' responses. Thus, deductive and inductive steps are integrated throughout the interview. To this end, the interview is conceptualised as a dialogue between researcher and respondent using an interview guide merely to support the flow of the conversation. Questions encouraging narrative talks as well as spontaneous probes and enquiries are used to ensure openness and orientation towards the problem. In the case under study, this procedure enabled me to ascertain how the respondents make sense of their situation in German hospitals as well as their subjective view of the problem i.e. their perception and interpretation of their professional integration on-site.

Interview guide

As with the expert interviews, the PCIs conducted with the CEE migrant physicians were based on an interview guide. The guide was divided into the following seven thematic sections: migration decision covering the motivation to migrate as well as the application procedure (I), the first phase in the hospital including initial impressions as well as experienced incorporation measures (II), collaboration and interactions with regard to medical colleagues, other hospital staff, and patients (III), the perception of working conditions (IV), the perceived professional development and state of one's own establishment on-site (V), perceived possibilities of professional advancement on-site (VI), reflections on migration decision and present experiences as well as future plans (VII) (for full interview guide see attachment ii).

Again, the interview questions were developed based on general knowledge and preliminary readings, and were oriented towards the chronological steps of the respondents' migration process, but were handled flexibly during the interview. The interview started with an open question encouraging the interviewees to talk about their hitherto professional pathway, from their initial motivation to study medicine to how they got to migrate to Germany. This far-reaching and extensive start of the interview proved valuable to help the respondents to become familiar with the interview situation and eased their flow of words. Each further interview section was introduced by an open question. Several questions targeted at reflections and evaluations further ensured the generation of subjective interpretations. The generated narration was then followed up by further enquiries. Like in the case of the expert interviews, the interview questions for the PCI were discussed with my first supervisor and other research colleagues. Additionally, four pilot interviews were conducted in order to test the comprehensibility and the adequate phrasing of the questions, as suggested, for instance, by Przyborski and Wohlrab-Sahr (2009, p. 22). Based on these interviews, wordings of individual questions and in some cases their order was changed again. This applied, for instance, to the opening question of the second interview section asking about the respondents' initial phase in the hospital. After the pre-test interviews the wording altered from "When you think back to the time right upon arrival in this hospital, how did you experience this initial phase?" to "When you think back to the time right upon arrival in this hospital, how did you *feel* in this initial phase?" Changing the phrasing from an "experience question" to a "feelings question" (Patton, 2002, p. 348ff.), enabled the respondents to think themselves back into the situation. This enhanced the possibility that interviewees opened up and revealed deeper insights that went beyond a pure factual account of what was new for them in that situation. Additionally, questions encouraging reflection and evaluation contributed to the generation of such interpretative patterns. Finally, again an open question for further statements and comments ensured the consideration of the interviewees' subjective relevance structures.

Course of the interview

In contrast to the experts, the migrant physicians were not always very talkative and keen on sharing information. Some were rather reserved and restrained in talking about their experiences and many enquiries were needed to keep up the conversation and retrieve the desired knowledge. In particular, questions addressing the relationship to colleagues and nurses were often answered very briefly saying that everything works just fine. This might indeed be the case, but the volatility with which this was said could also imply difficulties. Reasons for why interviewees were reluctant to mention potential difficulties could be concerns about confidentiality, unease in remembering certain situations, or discomfort in admitting discrimination since this could be perceived as questioning their professional identity as well as the purpose of their presence on-site.

Furthermore, questions targeted at potential structural inequalities, for instance, with regard to working hours, salary etc. did not retrieve elaborate responses. Since these questions were answered in a very casual way, I do not suspect that they intended to hide actual inequalities, but indeed did not perceive any. The same applied to inequalities based on gender. Most of the respondents stated that they did not experience any difficulties, but hypothesised that this might play a role later, once they have completed residency and are looking for a job, or with regard to promotions to higher positions. The reason the interviewees gave for assumed difficulties was that employers would prefer male over female physicians due to pregnancy and the expectation that women would rather stay home or reduce working hours in order to take care of children. The reason for why female junior physicians did not experience inequalities based on gender, although the medical profession is known to be discriminatory in this respect (e.g. Heru, 2005), could be that physicians are still following a standardised path during the training period. Additionally, the stress of finding one's way in a new working environment could have also been so demanding that the respondents did not have the capacity to be sensitive to such incidences.

A last group of questions that did not produce extensive replies were those targeted at the migrant physicians' involvement in medical associations and unions representing medical doctors. Many interviewees had not even heard about, for instance, the *Marburger Bund*, or did not show any interest. This could partially be due to an insufficient information policy on the part of these organisations and the hospital. However, a reason given by some of the interviewees was the number of new and unfamiliar aspects that they had to deal with in their daily routine. They felt so overwhelmed that so far they did not have the capacity to learn about options of professional organisation.

The interviewees' German language skills varied greatly. Some migrant physicians had noticeable difficulties in expressing themselves in German. Nevertheless, comprehension problems were rare and could mostly be dealt with by inquiring and repeating, respectively, what had been said.

The interviews with the migrant doctors were conducted in most cases in a doctor's room after work, or a meeting room in the hospital. In one case the interview took place in a corridor of the hospital, which significantly lowered the quality of the recording. In two cases interviews were conducted in the physicians' private apartments. The interviews lasted between 38 and 103 minutes and had an average length of about 60 minutes. Again, before starting the interview the respondents were informed about content and procedure and asked to sign a form confirming their consent to recording the interview and using the gained interview material. Directly after the interviews I wrote a postscript making notes about the interview situation, the impression I gained from the respondents as well as other observations, ideas, and remarks. These served the purpose of retaining the personal impression I had gained of the interviewee. Later on, these postscripts helped me with the interpretation of the interviews in terms of being able to better classify and understand certain statements based on the respondents' bearing during the interview. Altogether 21 PCIs with CEE migrant physicians were conducted in the time between November 2012 and April 2013.

4.3 Case selection and description of the sample

4.3.1   Case selection

CEE medical doctors were chosen as, to date, they form the biggest group of migrant physicians out of the EU member countries in German hospitals. Moreover, they are of special interest as they reflect the currently changing character of East-West migration. With *change*, I refer to their level of skill as well as their direct placement in the primary labour market on the one hand, and the demand-driven character of that migration on the other. It also considers the only recently granted freedom of movement and Germany's hitherto restrictive way of treating CEE immigrants.

As common in qualitative research, what Bryman (2012) terms a "generic purposive sampling" approach was applied looking for cases that "are relevant for the research questions" (ibid., p. 422). Hence, a strategic way of sampling was chosen that included two different levels – contexts and participants (ibid., p. 417f.). First of all, the contexts, i.e. the hospitals were chosen that were located in different parts of Germany as well as in cities and towns that differed in size. Contacts were established through directly approaching hospital administrations via phone or email. The contacted hospitals were chosen due to their location in a certain area, or based on specific recommendations of HR managers I had met at a relevant event connected to my topic of research. One such recommendation resulted in an invitation to a meeting of HR managers of different hospitals held by one hospital provider. In another case, a newspaper article on the situation with migrant physicians working on-site drew my attention to one of the facilities. Secondly, the interviewees were sampled. While the participants in the expert interviews, namely HR managers and medical directors, were given by definition, CEE physicians were sampled by a form of secondary selection (Morse, 1994, p. 228f.), i.e. through the distribution of requests for interviews including demographic questionnaires (see attachment iii). Based on these questionnaires the actual interviewees were to be sampled. Unfortunately, the requests could not be handed out to the migrant physicians directly. Due to matters of data protection the hospital administration could not provide me with the respective names or addresses. Therefore, in most cases the calls were distributed with the help of the hospital management or HR managers of the respective hospitals. For some of the contact persons, acting as a gatekeeper was in their own interest. The prospect of an evaluation of the situation of the respective physicians in their hospital played a decisive role for their agreement. Indeed, feedback regarding the overall findings of the study was offered. However, in order to counteract the notion of collaboration with the hospital administration on the part of the migrant doctors, the calls included a letter stating purpose and goal of the interviews and a guarantee that all information would be treated anonymously.

Due to the secondary selection of interviewees, the sample was heavily dependent on the accessibility of these CEE physicians in terms of readiness and willingness to be interviewed (Merkens, 2009, p. 288). Therefore, additional interviewees were recruited through snowball sampling, both within one hospital and across hospitals. This had the advantage of access to respondents that had not initially replied to the call, but could be motivated by their colleagues, friends or partners to do so. However, this procedure always bears the danger of the respective respondents talking about the content of the interview beforehand, which might influence the given answers. Additionally, it is natural that respondents recommend friends and colleagues that share certain sociodemographic characteristics and stances. Thus, the risk is to remain in similar networks, and to be limited in researching the full range of the field (Przyborski & Wohlrab-Sahr, 2009, p. 180). Consequently, I might not have had the chance to speak to migrant physicians from other countries beyond those represented in the sample, or of a different age and family status, who would have enabled me to gain a broader understanding of the research subject.

Some criteria had been appointed prior to sampling in order to guarantee representation as regards to content ("inhaltliche Repräsentanz") rather than a representative level as applied in quantitative research (Przyborski & Wohlrab-Sahr, 2009, p. 173f.). Hence, appointed criteria were that participants held the citizenship of one of the CEE EU member countries of the accession rounds 2004 and 2007, and that they had finished their medical studies outside Germany. The latter question was included due to previous research showing that employment in the German labour market was easier for migrants with German certificates compared to those with certificates from their home countries (Nohl, Schittenhelm, et al., 2010b). Moreover, both male and female physicians were included in order to provide for the lack of research on female highly skilled migrants (see e.g. Kofman, 2000).

Hence, the sample was stratified according to nationality, country of origin, and graduation from university, respectively, and gender. The initial criterion of immigration after the EU accession of the state of origin was given up during the process of data collection, since physicians who migrated as non-EU citizen represented valuable contrasting cases to illustrate changes regarding bureaucratic procedures to obtain the medical license.

4.3.2   Description of the sample

All interviewees in the sample were guaranteed full anonymity. To this end, names of the individual respondents and of hospitals, as well as locations, were replaced by pseudonyms, or circumscriptions. I refer to the experts using their professional title. For the migrant doctors, I chose names of physicians from US-American and German TV shows as pseudonyms. These pseudonyms were selected randomly and do not inform in any way about the respective migrant doctors' personality, age, specialisation or any other personal or professional features. By using these pseudonyms, I mainly intend to disguise the physicians' nationality. This is done due to the risk that in such a small overall sample, and particularly due to the small number of physicians who I interviewed in the different hospitals, their anonymity could not be maintained towards others working in the same hospital. Since hardly any significant, country-specific differences were observed, this does not pose a limitation to the presentation of the findings of the study.

Regarding the locations or the medical associations of a certain Land mentioned in the interviews, I chose to circumscribe them by referring, for instance, to "the hospital in [her home country]", or "[the responsible] medical association." The specific hospitals are referred to below with the letters A to G. However, in the presentation of the findings, they are referred to by indicating their size and location, for instance, as "city hospital" versus "rural hospital", or "small hospital in a rural area."

Hospitals

On the context-level, the sample consists of seven different hospitals located in four different Laender in the North, East, and West of Germany.[16] The two hospitals located in the East of Germany, on the territory of the former GDR, were located close to the Polish and Czech border respectively. The locations of all hospitals ranged in size from big cities to towns and small towns[17]. All in all, four hospitals were chosen that were located in a big city in the North, and one in the immediate surroundings of a big city in West Germany. Another hospital was located in a town in East Germany, and one in a town in West Germany. Additionally, one hospital was located in a small town in the East. All hospitals, apart from the three city hospitals in Northern Germany, were located in rural areas.

Apart from the size of the location, also the size of the chosen hospitals differed. Applying the measuring unit introduced above (ch. 2.2), two of the

16   For reasons of guaranteed anonymity, the precise locations will not be mentioned.
17   Big city – term used for cities of more than 100.000; town – term used for places of 20.000-100.000 inhabitants; small town – term used for places of 5.000-20.000 inhabitants as defined by Hass and Neumair (n.d.).

city hospitals in Northern Germany fell in the category of hospitals with more than 600 beds. All remaining hospitals fell in the category of 300-599 beds. Only the hospital in the small town in Eastern Germany fell in the category of 50-299 beds.

The different hospitals were held by different hospital providers, ranging from public to private non-profit, and private for-profit organisations. However, irrespective of the type of ownership, all hospitals that are "accredited in public hospital plans, meaning that they are considered to be necessary to provide equal and nationwide access to hospital care, are eligible for public funds" (Klenk & Pieper, 2013). Health insurances cover the operating costs, whereas the owner, i.e. the land, the private provider, or welfare organisation, respectively, covers the investment costs. Hence, the hospitals do not differ with regard to the socio-economic background of the patients.

Table 2 List of Hospitals

Hospital	Region	Location	Hospital size	Hospital provider
A	Eastern Germany	Small town	50-299 beds	Private non-profit
B	Eastern Germany	Town	300-599 beds	Private for-profit
C	Northern Germany	Big city	over 600 beds	Public
D	Northern Germany	Big city	over 600 beds	Public
E	Northern Germany	Big city	300-599 beds	Private non-profit
F	Western Germany	Suburb of big city	300-599 beds	Private non-profit
G	Western Germany	Town	300-599 beds	Private non-profit

Source: Own table

Experts

On the second level of sampling, the participants for the interviews were chosen. As outlined above, the experts who were interviewed were basically given by definition. However, both the HR manager and the medical director were not at my disposal in all hospitals. In one hospital, the one with less than 300 beds, I only spoke to the managing director who had human resource responsibility since the hospital neither employed a HR manager, nor a medical director. In the two biggest city hospitals, I only spoke to the respective medical directors, as the HR managers were too restrained for time. In the third city hospital, I only interviewed the HR manager, as no medical director was in office. The same applied to the hospital in a Western German town. However, here the reasons were again time constraints on behalf of the medical director. Finally, both the medical director and HR manager were at my disposal in the hospital in the town in Eastern Germany, as well as in the one in the suburb of a big city in Western Germany. The medical director was employed full time in only one of the two big city hospitals. All other medical directors that I interviewed were practicing medicine at the same time and filling the position on a voluntary basis. In one hospital, the interview started out with the HR manager and a personnel officer at the same time. However, after a short time the former had to leave for another appointment and the interview was continued with the personnel officer, only.

Table 3 List of Experts

Hospital	Professional title of expert(s) interviewed
A	managing director
B	human resource manager
	personnel officer
	medical director
C	medical director
D	medical director
E	human resource manager
F	human resource manager
	medical director
G	human resource manager

Source: Own table

Migrant physicians

The sample of the participants in the PCIs consisted of 21 CEE migrant physicians. Not all of the Eastern EU member states were covered. Participants came from seven different CEE states, namely Bulgaria (2 physicians), the Czech Republic (1 physician), Hungary (4 physicians), Lithuania (1 physician), Poland (3 physicians), Romania (8 physicians), and Slovakia (2 physicians). 13 of them were female and eight male. Upon their arrival in Germany about half of them were in their late 20s, the other half's age ranged from 31-40. Only five physicians in the sample arrived in Germany before or in the exact year of the accession of their home country to the EU.

Apart from two of the physicians who had completed their studies in a CEE country other than their home country, all had finished their medical studies in their home countries. Some had migrated to Germany immediately after graduation from university, while others had started residency in their home countries, or had worked abroad prior to going to Germany. One physician had started residency in a CEE country other than their country of origin. Only two out of 21 doctors arrived in Germany after having completed residency in order to then work in the same specialist field. Others who had already started, or even finished residency before migrating, either planned to continue residency in the same field, or opted for a different field, and thus started anew. Three of the physicians interviewed had already changed the hospital within Germany.

Again, they either continued their residency after this change, or opted for a different field of specialisation. Accordingly, at the time of the interviews, most of the physicians were employed as junior physicians in residency. Only three physicians in the sample were senior physicians (1 female, 2 male).

Table 4 List of Migrant physicians

Interview partner (IP)	pseudonym	gender	age (at time of interview)	children	year of arrival in GER	Position (physician)	family status
01	Dr Christa Brinkmann	f	35	yes	2009	Junior	married
02	Dr Roland Heilmann	m	40	yes	2004	Senior	married
03	Dr Mark Greene	m	26		2012	Junior	single
04	Dr Susan Lewis	f	27		2012	Junior	single
05	Dr Kathrin Globisch	f	25		2012	Junior	single
07	Dr Gregory House	m	28		2011	Junior	single
08	Dr Martin Stein	m	36		2008	Junior	single
09	Dr Elena Eichhorn	f	39	yes	2001	Senior	married
10	Dr Lea Peters	f	27		2011	Junior	single
14	Dr Meredith Grey	f	27		2011	Junior	single
17	Dr Doug Ross	m	33	yes	2007	Junior	married
18	Dr Christina Yang	f	37		2010	Junior	married
19	Dr Miranda Bailey	f	26		2011	Junior	single
21	Dr Niklas Ahrend	m	38	yes	2007	Senior	married
20	Dr Matteo Moreau	m	34	yes	2006	Junior	married
23	Dr Michaela Quinn	f	31	yes	2012	Junior	married
24	Dr Leyla Sherbaz	f	28		2012	Junior	single
25	Dr Karin Patzelt	f	27		2012	Junior	single
28	Dr Elias Bähr	m	32		2012	Junior	single
29	Dr Julia Berger	f	27		2012	Junior	single
30	Dr Theresa Koshka	f	31		2013	Junior	single

Source: Own table

The physicians in the sample specialised in different medical fields. Six physicians specialised in internal medicine (4 female, 2 male), three of them with the aim to become cardiologists later on (1 female, 2 male), and one of them with the aim to further specialise in gastroenterology (female). Four physicians specialised in anaesthesia (3 female, 1 male), three in vascular surgery (2 female, 1 male), two in neurology (1 female, 1 male), two in ear, nose and throat (ENT) medicine (male), one in orthopaedics (male), one in gynaecology (female), one in psychiatry (female), and one in haematology/oncology (female).

At least half of the physicians interviewed migrated together with their partners, or were joined by their partners – in the same location or elsewhere

81

in Germany – later on. In five cases, the partner also practiced medicine. Three out of the 13 female physicians in the sample had children who had all been born already before the interviewees had started or continued their residency in Germany. Four out of the eight male physicians were fathers. Most of their children had been born during their residency.

4.4 Data analysis

The first step to data analysis is the transcription of the recorded interview material. All interviews were transcribed verbatim and are available as word files. The 16 interviews that were conducted in the end of 2012 were transcribed by myself, whereas the remaining 14 interviews conducted in the beginning of 2013 were transcribed by a student assistant (see attachment iv for the transcription rules). Both the expert interviews and the PCIs were analysed with the help of the computer software MAXQDA.

4.4.1   Analysing the expert interviews

The material gained from the expert interviews is strongly structured due to the interview guide and the chronological inquiring of the separate steps of the recruitment process. It provides facts about how the recruitment takes places, which strategies are applied to attract CEE migrant physicians, and which measures are taken on the part of the hospital to incorporate the physicians. Correspondingly, an analytical procedure targeted at retrieving pure information seems suitable (Bogner et al., 2014, p. 72). Moreover, the posed questions for evaluation and reflection generated interpretative patterns that also have to be analysed. Thus, a method of data analysis is needed giving room for interpretation. To this end, a method combining deductive and inductive codes as described by Kelle and Kluge (2010) is applied. They suggest the usage of deductive heuristics as categories in order to construct a coding system. These deductive categories will then be inductively filled with empirical data (ibid., p. 63). Such heuristics can consist of abstract and empirically empty theoretical concepts, empirically empty categories of everyday knowledge such as those often used for the construction of the interview guide, and empirically substantial ("gehaltvoll") theoretical concepts (ibid., p. 62). In the present case, the empirically empty concepts derived from everyday knowledge used in the interview guide were employed to structure the coding scheme for the expert interviews. This was the case for the main categories *Reasons for recruitment*, *Reasons for recruitment from CEE*, *Recruitment strategies*, *Employment crite-*

ria, Support in initial phase, the broad category *Experiences, Challenges, Difficulties, Taking stock*, and *Future perspectives*. However, despite integration of prior knowledge, the challenge is to remain open for content and relevance structures emerging from the data. Therefore, these deductively derived code categories are completed with inductive categories. This applied for the category *Reasons for the shortage of physicians* which became relevant due to the fact that all of the interviewees named a perceived shortage of physicians as a reason for the recruitment and employment of migrant physicians and elaborated on the reasons thereof.

After a first cycle of coding in which test passages were broadly coded with these main categories, only those categories and text passages were considered for a second coding cycle that were regarded as productive and relevant to answer the research questions. For example interview questions about human resource strategies posed to the HR managers in the sample did not prove pertinent for the specific case of the professional integration of migrant physicians as these were rather broad and targeted at the entire medical work force on-site. Hence, the respective deductive coding category was moved under a category called "miscellaneous" and not further considered.

The remaining main categories were then completed with sub codes further specifying the content with the help of different dimensions of these categories. Again, these sub codes were partly derived deductively, and partly inductively through the comparison of the different text passages that were assigned to a main category (ibid., p. 76). For example, for code *Support in initial phase*, the sub codes *Professional incorporation* and *Linguistic incorporation* were determined, matching the respective interview questions. Additionally, a third sub code emerged from the data, namely, sub code *practical support* including respective measures that were provided on the part of hospitals. While the latter code was derived from factual information provided by the respondents, other text passages required more interpretation to be summarised in sub codes. This was the case for those completing the main code *Taking stock*. Passages ascribed to this category were derived from questions encouraging reflection and evaluation. Hence sub codes such as *Migrant physicians as inevitable necessity* and *Migrant physicians as enrichment* were derived purely inductively. Also all additional codes filling the deductively set sub codes, such as the code *Support with flat hunting* and code *Provision of accommodation upon arrival* were derived purely inductively from the data filling up the grid with empirical material and concepts related to the subject ("gegenstandsbezogen").

4.4.2   Analysing the PCIs

The PCIs with the CEE migrant physicians formed the focal point of the study. In contrast to the expert interviews, the focus of these interviews was only partly on the procedural knowledge describing the migration process, but mainly on the interpretative knowledge in terms of how the migrant doctors subjectively make sense of the situation, which meaning they attribute to their migration and their experiences on-site, how they perceive the problem under study, and which action logics they develop based on this perception. Nevertheless, since the PCIs also produced different forms of knowledge, different coding steps were applied in order to fully exploit the informational content of the data.

In a first step, I indexed the entire interview material and categorised it by keywords with general thematic codes indicating the subject of the passage (Saldaña, 2013, p. 88). In many cases these would match the different sections of the interview guide, such as *Migration motives, Migration strategies, Experiences and challenges* and so on. Based on these descriptive codes, again, text passages were put aside that were found to be less relevant for answering research questions and those which did not yield useful information, such as those targeted at the migrant doctors' involvement in professional organisations. In a first cycle of coding the remaining passages were then initially coded examining nuances and variations within the broader categories through comparison (ibid., p. 100) in order to become familiar with the material. To this end, different coding techniques were applied. Additional codes were employed representing the content of the coded text passage; these included *process codes* that focused on actions and were intended to capture ways of dealing with certain problems (ibid., p. 96). Correspondingly, these proved useful, for example, to filter out different steps the respondents described with respect to their migration strategies, or coping strategies physicians applied in response to challenges and barriers they were confronted with. Moreover, *value codes* targeted at values, attitudes and beliefs and helping to retrieve perceptions and evaluations expressed by the interviewees were applied (ibid., p. 110ff.). Another employed coding technique during this first cycle of coding was *versus coding* which is used to identify competing goals and interests, as well as conflicts (ibid., p. 115). In the present case these proved useful to identify, for example, comparisons between host and home countries, but also conflicts described between the physicians and other actors involved. While the first interview transcripts were coded line-by-line in order to employ the greatest possible openness and explore the material, in the course of the process the coded passages became more extensive as I was able to draw on previously assigned codes.

In a second coding cycle, some of the initial codes were taken to a more conceptual level, whereas others that were rather classificatory or indexical in character remained this way. The latter applied, for instance, to those codes depicting the migration motives (e.g. *professional reasons* or *financial reasons*), and those representing the migration strategy the migrant physicians had chosen (e.g. *approached agency directly* or *contact to hospital on job fair*). Codes that were applied to text passages containing interpretative knowledge had to be further analysed in order to get to the underlying, subjective understanding of the problem and relevance structures. Accordingly, a method of data analysis was required that enables the reconstruction of the meaning attached to the phenomenon, and to generate concepts capturing the identified aspects of the phenomenon. For this purpose, the three-step coding technique of the Grounded Theory Methodology was employed (Strauss & Corbin, 1991). Therefore, the initial codes that had been assigned during "open coding" were condensed into broader categories and subcategories. For instance, all aspects of the professional routine that the interviewees had described as hampering the application of their professional skills and knowledge were subsumed under the concept *barrier to transfer of professional qualifications*. In a second step called "axial coding" these individual aspects were compared with each other in order to identify similarities and define the context, properties, and dimensions of found categories. Hence, these were refined using more specific categories such as *lack of institutional knowledge* or *inter-professional struggles* with several subcategories. In the case of *inter-professional struggles* these were, for instance, d*evaluation of cultural capital due to inexperience*, *devaluation of cultural capital due to language deficits*, or *devaluation of cultural capital due to deviation from routine*. Like these examples show, in this step I also integrated theoretical concepts from the literature which were found in the data such as "cultural capital" (Bourdieu, 1984), or also "Kompetenzdarstellungskompetenz" ("competence to represent competence") (Pfadenhauer, 2003).

In a third step, "selective coding", the categories were set in relation to each other and incorporated into key categories on a more abstract level. This way, for instance, I used the key category *loss of status* to bring together the various barriers migrant physicians encountered, and their perception of these incidences.

4.5 Critical reflection on biases and methodical shortcomings

A number of methodical limitations to the study can be identified. Due to issues of data protection, in many cases it was not possible to approach the migrant physicians directly. Instead they had to be sampled through the respective hospital administrations. That way, the respondents might have felt less free in their responses and elaborations during the interviews. They might have been suspicious that their superiors would learn about their statements, and might have thus been restrained in their responses. Moreover, this way of sampling might have kept others from participating in the study completely. In order to counteract such incidents, confidentiality and anonymity were assured in both the interview request as well as immediately before starting the interview. Nevertheless, remaining insecurities on the part of the migrant doctors in this respect cannot fully be ruled out. Hence, I might not have been able to speak to migrant physicians who experienced major difficulties in the hospital, but were afraid that the information they share, or their identity would not be kept confidential.

However, due to this procedure the received sample is partially clustered (Merkens, 2009, p. 293) as these interviewees knew each other and hence shared similar experiences, had the same specialisation, or even worked on the same ward. This obviously bears the risk that respondents exchanged information about the subject of the interviews which might have affected the individual responses (Przyborski & Wohlrab-Sahr, 2009, p. 180). Nevertheless, this procedure did not impair the outcome of the interviews as it was only applied in a supplementary manner and thus to a very limited degree. Moreover, the initial criteria that were established a priori also remained valid with regard to those participants.

The fact that I as a member of the German majority society conducted the interviews asking about experiences in exactly this society might have additionally impaired the interviewees' response behaviour, since I might have been "perceived as an outsider" (Rubin & Rubin, 2012, p. 182). That might have had the effect that, "[i]nstead of answering questions from their own experience, the interviewees answer with what they think is the appropriate cultural response" (ibid.), or is appropriate in terms of social desirability. The different cultural background and related cultural modes and codes of conduct of interviewer and interviewee is, however, not only crucial due to a different socialisation in terms of different countries of origin, but also in terms of different professional fields (Kelle & Kluge, 2010, p. 34). Not having any medical training, I lack an understanding of cultural and linguistic codes as well as patterns of interpretation prevalent in the medical field. "Control interviews" with two German physicians employing the same interview guide as for the migrant physicians were conducted to avoid misunderstandings in this respect. From these I gained additional information, such as the fact that the relationship between inexperienced junior physicians and nurses is in general tense at the beginning, irrespective of a status as migrant. Moreover, findings were discussed with practitioners in hospitals, as well as with other researchers in the field in order to arrive at a deeper understanding thereof. Of particular help was the exchange with Polish research colleagues at the Centre of Migration Research in Warsaw, Poland who had conducted research on medical migration from Poland previously, and shared their interpretations of the material with me. For instance, I learnt that in Poland physicians tend to not explain medical procedures very extensively to their patients. Such insights provided me with useful background knowledge for understanding certain difficulties Polish physicians encountered in German hospitals. Nevertheless, this was just one national perspective out of seven represented in the sample. Hence, again the problem could not be excluded entirely.

Furthermore, the fact that the interviews were conducted in German, which was not the respondents' native language, might have had an impact. The interviewees might have felt insecure and limited in how to express themselves due to linguistic weaknesses, which might have altered their statements. Again, misunderstandings might have occurred based on the unfamiliarity of me as interviewer with the respective native languages that might have informed their choice of words and formulations when expressing themselves in German. Hence, I might have missed crucial subtleties (Rubin & Rubin, 2012, p. 186). Nonetheless, since no linguistic analysis is conducted, these shortcomings are expected to not restrict the validity of the data.

A last aspect refers to the process of coding and analysing the data. In order to limit the subjectivity in the interpretation of the data, it is recommended to establish an inter-coder reliability by analysing the data together with other researchers (Bryman, 2012, p. 304). Since in my case this was not possible, I tried to reduce the resulting limitations with regard to the validity of the findings by discussing the identified codes and concepts at various stages of the analysis with my supervisors, and by repeatedly presenting my findings to them and other research colleagues, e.g. in method courses and workshops on coding and data analysis.

5 Managing the shortage of physicians – institutional strategies in the recruitment of migrant physicians

Subsequent to the presentation of the research design and methods, chapters 5 and 6 detail the empirical findings of the study. Chapter 5 covers the perspective of the HR managers and medical directors of the respective hospitals based on the conducted expert interviews. It depicts the recruitment procedure and thus sets the institutional frame for the professional integration, and perceptions, of the CEE migrant physicians. Additionally, it reflects its assessment by relevant actors involved on the receiving side of the migration. The chapter first depicts the HR managers' and medical directors' explanations about why their hospitals rely on migrant physicians (5.1.). Second, it describes the applied recruitment strategies (5.2), before outlining experienced challenges with – and resulting criteria for – the recruitment of CEE migrant physicians (5.3). The following section describes the measures taken on the part of the hospital administrations in order to induct and bind the migrant physicians into the daily routine of each respective hospital (5.4). Finally, the last two sections provide an evaluation of the situation and future considerations by the HR managers and medical directors (5.5), followed by the presentation of interim conclusions (5.6).

5.1 "Don't know where our medical students remain – they don't apply to us"[18] [19]

When questioned why migrant physicians are employed, the HR managers and medical directors in the sample mainly referred to increasing difficulties they experienced in filling their vacancies with German (-trained)[20] medical staff (e.g. IP11: 9; IP12: 6; IP26: 8). However, there are different degrees of staff shortages in the different hospitals. In the early 2000s, rural hospitals[21] in Eastern and Western Germany already struggled with a staffing problem (IP06: 8; IP26: 10), while the representatives of the city hospitals stated that they are

18 „Weiß nicht, wo unsere Medizinstudenten bleiben - bei uns bewerben sie sich nicht" (IP12: 6).
19 All interviews were conducted in German and translated into English by myself with the help of Anissa Kirchner and Eva Loy.
20 With the term "German (-trained) physician/doctor", I refer to Germans and non-Germans who have completed medical studies at a German university, in contrast to "migrant physicians/doctors" who have completed studies abroad.
21 To simplify matters, I refer to the hospitals in the sample as "rural" and "city hospitals", respectively, in the presentation and discussion of the empirical findings. However, I do not claim generalisation of the findings for all rural and city hospitals in Germany.

occasionally affected by staffing issues in recent years before the 2012 and 2013 interviews (IP15: 10; IP22: 20). Unlike the rural hospitals, the presence of migrant physicians was not a new phenomenon to the city hospitals. However, the motivation for migrant physician employment, and where the majority originated from had changed.

The reason for this recent change in at least two of the city hospitals that function as training hospitals for a medical school nearby was the loss of a particular group of migrant physicians. These hospitals provided educational endowment for medical graduates mainly from countries such as Syria and Libya. These non-EU physicians were funded through a stipend provided by their respective embassies and completed for residency as guest physicians on-site. However, due to legal changes, specialist training was no longer possible in a German hospital without being officially employed by the facility. Thus, the bureaucratic procedure for non-EU physicians to complete residency on-site became more complicated due to the required equivalency tests. Moreover, the hospital could not offer many additional official positions, so that this option was no longer available to the same extent. The medical director of one of the city hospitals with more than 600 beds explained his hospital had shifted from being in strong demand as site for specialist training by international medical graduates, to depending more and more on migrant physicians for basic operation, as the loss of this one group coincided with the decline in applications from German (-trained) physicians that other facilities had suffered from already earlier (IP16: 6/8). Consequently, the employment of migrant physicians had become more urgent for the city hospitals.

The reasons that the respondents identified for causing the perceived shortage of German (-trained) physicians corresponded to those given in the literature and discussed above (see ch. 2.2.1). They referred to structural changes in the organisation of health care in German hospitals, and to changes with respect to preferences and attitudes of young generations of physicians. All these developments were identified as most pronounced in rural hospitals, and required ever greater numbers of medical staff in order to cover the overall work load. However, the desired measures taken by the German government to address the problem failed to appear, to the dismay of HR managers and medical directors.

Regarding structural changes, the interviewees described how new scientific knowledge and developments lead to an increase of possibilities for medical treatments in terms of surgery and examination procedures accompanied by a higher demand for medical treatment on the part of patients (IP27: 76). Additionally, the differentiation of medical fields into an ever increasing number of sub-specialisations (IP06: 6), and the change in work time regulations after the verdict of the ECJ in 2003 enacting that physicians are not allowed to work at the day after having completed a night shift (IP27: 76), contributed to the extension of staff appointment schemes. The extent of this development was illustrated by one medical director who stated: "When I started we had eight physicians in internal medicine, now there are 25" (IP27: 72).[22] Hence, developments within the organisation and provision of medical care were identified as increasing a general demand of medical personnel.

According to the respondents, the situation was further amplified by major losses in the medical work force related to a change in professional attitudes across the generations. They named an imminent drop-out of a numerically strong generation of physicians (IP11: 61), as well as an increasing number of medical students not finishing their studies (IP06: 6), and medical graduates leaving the profession as causing the losses. The latter find employment in non-curative medical fields such as the pharmaceutical industry, in hospital administrations, and health insurances (e.g. IP06: 6; IP22: 137, IP26: 54), or emigrate in order to practice medicine abroad (e.g. IP16: 84; IP22: 137). The interviewees accorded that emigration was not the dominating factor, as the actual numbers of those leaving the country fell below estimates (IP27: 74), and many would return to Germany after some time abroad (IP26: 54). However, observed emigration contributed to their assumption that dissatisfaction with the local working conditions was the driving force for drop-outs. In this respect, they identified a generational change among physicians. While older generations of doctors would have dedicated large parts of their free time to their profession, the younger cohorts – often described as 'generation Y' – would attribute more meaning to their 'work-life-balance.' Members of this generation were said to give priority to leisure time and family over having a career. Older interviewees especially described this trend as problematic due to an increasing demand of physicians and perceived declining quality of their training.

Generation Y, a very big problem, a massive problem. (…) That's of course completely different and we've to respond to that and there are people, they say in the future we'll need two and a half doctors for what one's doing today. (…) So, that's something that's making us older people worry, because the attendance time is not only time in which you are away from your family – that is what it is often presented like nowadays – but attendance time is also a time to gain a lot of experience (IP11: 63/65).[23]

This development does not only mark a change in the self-perception of physicians as a professional group, but also provokes the concern that this attitude, again, might augment the demand of physicians. Yet, the fear of an enlarged

---

22   „[IA]ls ich anfing hatten wir in der Inneren Abteilung acht Ärzte und jetzt sind es 25" (IP27: 72).

23   „Generation Y, ein ganz großes Problem, ganz riesiges Problem. (…) [D]as ist natürlich schon wirklich ganz anders, und darauf müssen wir uns auch einstellen und da gibt es Leute, die sagen, in Zukunft brauchen wir für das, was heute ein Arzt macht, zweieinhalb. (…) Also das ist etwas, was uns Älteren große Sorgen macht, weil die Anwesenheitszeit ist nicht nur eine Zeit, in der man von der Familie fern ist – so wird das ja heute oftmals dargestellt – sondern Anwesenheitszeit ist auch eine Zeit, in der man viele Erfahrungen macht" (IP11: 63/65).

demand of part-time arrangements was even more focussed on female physicians. Since their share had risen tremendously within recent years (see ch. 2.2.3), HR managers and medical directors anticipated a steeper shortage of medical doctors. This concern was founded in the assumption that female physicians would drop out of their professional activity temporarily, and would tend to prefer reduced working hours when rearing children (e.g. IP16: 80; IP22: 137; IP26: 55).

The rural hospitals in the sample were affected by the perceived shortage of physicians to a larger degree than the city hospitals. The HR managers and medical directors identified the cause to be the unattractive rural locales for young physicians. Small towns, far away from medical schools were said to be less popular for medical graduates who would prefer living in urban areas, as well as staying within or at least close to their place of study (IP11: 10).

So, this internal maelstrom of positions for physicians through the expansion of staff appointment schemes in each hospital is creating a shortage. And the central hospitals, especially in university cities, they can suck up the students, because there they like to stay there and in the rural areas, they've the difficulties, of course (IP27: 72).[24]

Hence, interviewees saw the changes discussed above as being amplified and most pronounced in rural facilities due to the unpopularity of the small hospital's remote locations.

Vis-à-vis this situation, HR managers and medical directors identified shortages as "a clearly political issue" (IP06: 6, see also IP16: 80)[25], and saw the German government responsible to find a solution. They acknowledged an increase in the number of medical graduates as one solution in the hopes that market would regulate supply and demand and equilibrate distribution of physicians across all hospitals in the country. Consequently, they requested political measures to increase the number of university places for medicine (e.g. IP22: 137; IP27: 72), and lower the high entrance requirements for medical studies (IP26: 54; IP31: 115). Yet, political measures have fallen short. Given the fact that the completion of the professional training of physicians takes about 15 years, respondents gave rise to the concern, that an increase of university places would show its effect, in any case, only in the future (IP11: 61). The paradoxical situation of German students going abroad in order to study medicine because they do not meet the entrance requirements at German universities, or engaging in law suits to fight for places to study in Germany, caused further dissatisfaction.

---

24   „Also dieser innere Sog an Arztstellen durch Ausweitung der Stellenpläne in jedem Krankenhaus, der macht natürlich dann einen Mangel. Und die Krankenhäuser die zentral liegen, besonders in Universitätsstädten, die können sich vollsaugen, weil die [Studierenden] da gerne bleiben und die in der Peripherie, die haben natürlich Schwierigkeiten" (IP27: 72).

25   „eine klare politische Sache" (IP06: 6;)

And it would require a tremendous step to stop this... (...) At the moment they're fighting for one place to study more or less in court. But we don't need one place more or less, we surely need more than thousand more or less (IP11: 63).[26]

This inactivity of the German government vis-à-vis the urgency of the situation was incomprehensible to the interviewees who expressed the suspicion that the German government was keen to cut costs for medical training streamline the health care system, describing this behaviour as "artificial shortage" (IP06: 87)[27]. They suspected that the government aimed to reduce the overall number of hospitals with the help of increased competitive conditions due to a shortage of doctors.

In my opinion this is clearly politics. Yes, from the perspective of politicians there are way too many hospitals and because of that they won't do anything. They let the hospital fight for their existence and this causes a natural selection. And then they slowly start introducing new laws (IP31: 117).[28]

Therefore, HR managers and medical directors perceived themselves as left alone by the German government. Facing a lack of applications to open medical positions and thus the risk of deficiencies in the provision of medical care, particularly those representing smaller hospitals felt constrained to find alternative solutions. The possibility they opted for was the recruitment of physicians from abroad. Due to major legal changes facilitating bureaucratic procedures for migrant physicians to obtain the German medical license (see ch. 2.2.3), this measure became even less complicated. However, the fact that barriers for migrant physicians to practice medicine in Germany were lowered was not accepted to be an adequate step to address the shortage. On the contrary, the dependence on migrant doctors was partially perceived as an "evidence for incapacity for Germany" (IP06: 6)[29].

In sum, the respondents identified the reasons for a greater demand of medical personnel as caused by structural developments in the organisation of medical care. While HR managers and medical directors of the city hospitals managed to escape the problem for some time, they found themselves confronted with the same difficulties their colleagues from rural hospitals experienced after the loss of the 'guest' physicians. In particular, the respondents representing rural hospitals demonstrated distrust toward the recruitment of

---

26 „Und es würde aber eines gewaltigen Schrittes bedürfen, um mit diesem, mit diesem Irrsinn Schluss zu machen. (...) Jetzt wird ja momentan vor Gericht gestritten, ob es einen Studienplatz mehr oder weniger gibt. Wir brauchen aber nicht einen Studienplatz mehr oder weniger, wir brauchen aber sicherlich mehrere tausend mehr oder weniger" (IP11: 63).

27 „Künstliche Verknappung" (IP06: 87).

28 „[M]einer Meinung [nach] ist das ganz klar Politik ja, wir haben nach der Meinung [der PolitikerInnen] viel zu viele Krankenhäuser und aufgrund der Sache halten die erst mal die Füße still. Die lassen sich erst mal die Häuser untereinander bekriegen, auffressen und dann findet da äh, äh, ja, eine natürliche Aussiebung statt und dann kann man irgendwann neue Gesetzgebung machen" (IP31: 117).

29 „Armutszeugnis für Deutschland" (IP06: 6).

migrant physicians, which can be interpreted as the self-perpetuating character of the medical profession on the one hand, and an overall averseness towards immigrants within the German society on the other. Regardless, it implies that HR managers and medical directors perceive themselves as victims of a situation which they cannot alter, but which they are forced to face. Hence, the undertaken employment of migrant physicians appears as reluctant mission in an otherwise hopeless situation.

5.2 "Employment agencies for physicians are a big business"[30]

Due to the lack of political action in the form hoped for by the HR managers and medical directors, they found themselves constrained to rely on migrant physicians. While the respondents from the rural hospitals stated CEE countries as main source for recruitment, in the city hospitals CEE physicians constituted one group among other migrant doctors, albeit their number is increasing. According to the degree of experienced shortage of physicians in the respective hospitals as depicted above (ch. 5.1), the respondents applied different recruitment strategies to fill their vacancies. While the city hospitals could widely rely on traditional measures, the rural hospitals had to engage in active recruitment from abroad. With 'active recruitment' I refer to recruitment strategies that are explicitly targeted at physician from abroad, such as employing recruitment agencies specialising in the field, or founding partnerships with medical schools in CEE countries. The following depiction of these strategies applies to both the recruitment of junior physicians in residency, and of medical specialists. Head physicians are excluded, since these were mainly sought by head hunters in German-speaking countries.

5.2.1   Traditional recruitment strategies

Location in bigger cities and ability to provide a wide range of opportunities for residency in a large spectrum of medical fields resulted in lower shortages in city hospitals and fewer difficulties in filling physician vacancies. Only individual departments had occasionally been affected. Contrary to rural hospitals, the city hospitals had not significantly changed their recruitment strategies in response to the increasing demand.

Particularly one of the city hospitals with more than 600 beds in the sample that functioned as training hospital for medical faculties nearby used to be able

---

30   „Ärztevermittlung ist ein großes Geschäft" (IP11: 19).

to mainly rely on unsolicited applications in order to fill its vacancies. Largely this was still the case, however, as outlined above, these unsolicited applications did not only stem from German (-trained) physicians, but also migrant physicians applied in that way (see ch. 6.1). In some cases, an intermediary level directed migrant medical doctors to the respective hospitals; namely, the Goethe institute where many migrant physicians take German classes and obtain their certificate of German proficiency. There, migrant physicians were provided with contacts of hospitals to apply to, as the responsible medical director explained: "The Goethe-Insitute functions as... not as an employment agency, but as supporting agency. They've the addresses of all hospitals and they pass them on" (IP15: 10-12).[31] Reason for these lucky circumstances were most likely the facility's size and its reputation as training hospital.

Nonetheless, as HR managers and medical directors stated, also in these city hospitals, difficulties in filling vacancies incrementally occurred. Unsolicited applications, especially of German (-trained) physicians, increasingly failed to appear. Therefore, the respondents had to publish job advertisements, as one of the medical directors explained,

From time to time we've these [job] advertisements when departments have difficulties to fill a vacancy. Then we've a certain budget which I manage as medical director. Since the shortage of physicians is increasing in Germany, one ad in the medical journal costs €10,000 and sometimes there is no response at all – also none within Germany. Sometimes we advertise in the medical journal or in internet journals, forums of professional journals for a certain cost contribution and then we wait for applications. But that's very difficult. And then we most of the time receive applications from Arabic States or Middle and Eastern Europe (IP15: 26).[32]

Traditional recruitment strategies did not solicit German (-trained) physicians anymore in the city hospital sample: the applications they received increasingly stemmed from migrant physicians.

---

31 „[D]as Goethe-Institut funktioniert quasi so als... (…). Ja nicht Stellenvermittler, aber äh, aber als Unterstützer. Die haben quasi von allen Kliniken und so Anschriften und dann ist das so Stille Post, ne" (IP15: 10-12).

32 „Wir haben teilweise die, diese Inserate, wenn Abteilungen Schwierigkeiten haben, Stellen zu besetzen. Dann haben wir ein bestimmtes Budget, das ich auch verwalte als ärztlicher Geschäftsführer, weil es so ist, dass der Ärztemangel natürlich sehr um sich greift in Deutschland und dann eine Anzeige im Ärzteblatt kostet 10000€ und manchmal ist da dann gar keine Resonanz, auch keine deutsche Resonanz darauf. Oder wir inserieren teilweise im Ärzteblatt oder in Internetmagazinen von Fachzeitschriften für einen bestimmten Kostenbeitrag und warten dann auf Bewerbungen. Was aber sehr schwierig ist. Und da bewerben sich meistens dann, also entweder aus arabischen Staaten oder aus Mittel- und Osteuropa" (IP15: 26).

5.2.2   Recruitment agencies

Another way for migrant physicians to make it into German hospitals was with the help of human resource agencies specialising in the recruitment of physicians. Although particularly respondents from urban hospitals stated their reluctance to cooperate with such agencies, both the city hospitals, as well as the rural hospitals in the sample relied on the services of recruitment agencies, at least in pressing situations. Since the beginning of the shortage of physicians in Germany in the early 2000s, an increasing number of such agencies, located in Germany as well as in the respective countries of origin, appeared on the market. Reacting to the growing demand they promoted the increase of migrant physicians in the German health care system.

We simply had to help ourselves somehow. And then in the end there were more and more international physicians on the market and the head hunters or employment agencies mushroomed and we were receiving more and more offers (IP26: 10).[33]

Agencies specialised in the recruitment of CEE physicians to German hospitals, and offered their services. However, the interviewees described a broad diversity among the large number of recruitment agencies of how they got in touch with their clients and of how they operated. Some of them approached hospitals on their own initiative, offering candidates to fill their vacancies either on an unsolicited basis, or in response to job advertisements published by the hospital. Others worked in a less ad-hoc manner and instead aimed at establishing a close cooperation with the respective hospital in order to serve their concrete needs. While HR managers and medical directors of city hospitals primarily had encounters with the former, small hospitals located in rather rural areas tended to rely on the latter. Again, this division reflects the degree to which the different hospitals suffered from unfilled vacancies.

Being able to rely on the fact that there were medical doctors – whether German (-trained) or not – willing to apply for an open position, the city hospitals did not have to contact a recruitment agency, at the time of the interview. Nevertheless, they were approached by agencies that the interviewees did not regard as trustworthy due to perceived discordance and lack of effort to appropriately place the physicians they represented. One HR manager illustrated:

A classic reaction towards each advertisement is that I talk only to agencies the day after publishing. They want to offer great physicians to me who coincidentally are [onsite] and coincidentally absolutely want to become orthopaedists or whatever we are looking for at the moment. [...] That's a little like wanting to sell a slave to me. They don't take care of anything. They call me two times and want an incredible amount of

---

33   „[W]ir mussten uns dann einfach irgendwo weiterhelfen. Und dann kam das letztendlich so, dass wirklich auch immer mehr ausländische Ärzte auf dem Markt erschienen, die Headhunter oder die Personalvermittlungsagenturen wie Pilze aus dem Boden schossen und immer mehr Angebote auch eigentlich rein kamen" (IP26: 10).

money for the negotiation. And I don't want to work with such people. I don't want that and as long as we don't have to I don't do that (IP22: 26-31).[34]

In general, interviewees were sceptical towards the recruitment agencies as well as their services. Other HR managers and medical directors also criticised the agencies' way of operating, and were suspicious of the quality of their services, but also of the qualifications of the physicians they wanted to place. Nevertheless, not all of the representatives of city hospitals had always been in the position to refrain from making use of the services offered by a recruitment agency.

So, especially from Romania I know one [agency] which offers their services again and again. They also send profiles of applicants. In principle they want 1-2 monthly salaries as a commission and then offer applicants. We sometimes hired them when we had a shortage (IP15: 28).[35]

Hence, in very pressing situations, also respondents representing city hospitals found themselves constrained to rely on an agency, nonetheless.

Representatives of the rural facilities, however, had to frequently rely on recruitment agencies, and recruited the majority of their medical staff that way in order to fill the vacancies in the hospital. No longer being able to fill their vacancies by own means, the HR managers and medical directors of the rural hospitals in the sample decided to engage in active recruitment from abroad. Rural HR managers were satisfied with the service of the recruitment agencies they consulted. However, they did not remain passive, but took the initiative and time to get to know different recruitment agencies, their philosophies and concepts, as well as their way of operating. Additionally, they negotiated conditions that suited them and tested their services, before engaging in a more stable cooperation. As a result, they established a close collaboration with an agency they trusted and that they approached whenever they had an open position. "So far this worked out excellently. So I sticked to it and I can say I don't even have a handful of agencies which we work with. Maximum three. Yes, now we're using these channels as well" (IP31: 13).[36]

34 „Klassisch ist die Reaktion auf jedes Inserat die, dass Tag eins nach Veröffentlichung daraus besteht, dass ich nur mit Agenturen spreche, die mir ganz tolle Ärzte andienen wollen, die zufällig gerade [vor Ort] sind und zufällig unbedingt Orthopäde oder was wir auch gerade suchen, werden wollen. Die wimmel ich aber alle ab, weil ich das Modell für ausgesprochen unseriös halte. (…) Das hat so ein bisschen was von Sklaven verkaufen. Die eh, kümmern sich um nichts. Die telefonieren dann zweimal mit mir und wollen dann unheimlich viel Geld für die Vermittlung haben. Und mit solchen Leuten möchte ich nicht zusammenarbeiten. (…) [D]as möchte ich nicht und solange wir nicht müssen, machen wir das auch nicht" (IP22: 26-31).

35 „Also gerade aus Rumänien weiß ich jetzt eine [Agentur], die immer wieder sich anbietet. Die auch Bewerberprofile schickt. Die wollen im Prinzip dann 1-2 Monatsgehälter als Provision haben und bieten Bewerber an. Wir haben teilweise die angestellt, wenn Mangel war" (IP15: 28).

36 „[D]as hat bis jetzt hervorragend geklappt. Dabei bin ich dann auch geblieben, also ich kann sagen ich habe noch nicht mal eine Handvoll Agenturen wo wir jetzt damit zusammenarbeiten. Also maximal drei. Ja, wo wir dann auch diese Kanäle jetzt nutzen" (IP31: 13).

Hence, instead of making a random choice, respondents who said to have a close cooperation with an agency undertook a very careful and considerate selection process in order to find a candidate who was motivated and who fit into the team. To this end, they invited potential candidates that got suggested by the recruitment agency for a job interview in order to get to know the physicians in person. Already on that occasion, some HR managers and medical directors offered the candidate work shadowing on-site. That way, the physicians had the chance to get to know the hospital in order to make an informed decision. At the same time, HR managers and medical directors had an opportunity to form an impression of respective candidates' character, motivation, and their German language proficiency (IP27: 30; IP31: 125).

Human resource agencies played a central role in the active and passive recruitment of migrant physicians. Even respondents who initially declared their suspicion and aversion towards these agencies had to admit that in pressing situations they had to rely on their services. This highlights the severity of physician shortages and also a lack of commitment to find trustworthy cooperation partners, and good medical personnel. Counter urban experience, rural HR managers' and medical directors' accounts demonstrate successful collaboration with recruitment agencies.

5.2.3   Partnerships with universities in CEE countries

Rural hospitals additionally solicited physicians from abroad through the establishment of partnerships between their hospital or hospital holder, respectively, and medical schools and faculties of universities in CEE countries, particularly in the Baltics or Poland. In the sample, this applied to one of the hospitals located in the border region in Eastern Germany, as well as two smaller hospitals located in rural areas in Western Germany held by the same hospital owner. The medical director of the former explained that in times of severe shortages they could rely on Polish physicians and medical graduates from a neighbouring Polish city:

The connections are getting closer and closer. We already train students from Poland and partly we also teach in Poland at the university. This shows how strongly the connection grows (IP11: 61). [37]

He stressed this as a locational advantage of his hospital, and was very much interested to further strengthen this relationship in the long term.

In Western Germany, rural facilities also established similar partnerships. Medical students from their partner universities in the Baltics came in order to

---

37   „Die Verbindungen werden immer enger. Wir bilden jetzt schon Studenten aus Polen [aus], zum Teil lehren wir auch in Polen, an der Hochschule. Also das ist sehr, sehr stark wie das zusammenwächst" (IP11: 61).

complete internships or their clinical traineeship in the German partner hospitals, getting a first insight into the hospital routine. The interviewees were greatly satisfied with this arrangement and hoped that these medical students would later decide to complete specialisation on-site, as one of the HR managers asserted:

That was great. They were extremely motivated, committed and their German was very structured, too. (…) And at the moment, actually in the last week, I've two who did their internship [in the other hospital I work at]. They would now like to start their specialist training here. So, we're also opening this channel currently, work strongly on it to acquire young university graduates from abroad (IP31: 13).[38]

The clear advantage for the hospital then would be that the young doctors already got a first impression of how a German hospital is organised and operates.

In sum, the recruitment strategies applied on the part of the respective HR managers and medical directors were demand-driven and primarily ad-hoc. However, there were major differences in strategies applied by those representing city hospitals and those representing more remotely located facilities. While the former relied on recruitment agencies only in cases of emergency when not having any applicants, the latter approached the problem in a more strategic and systematic way cooperating with agencies as well as with medical schools in CEE on a regular basis.

5.3 "We have to keep the business running"[39]

Albeit reluctantly in the case of the rural hospitals, and rather nonchalantly in the case of the city hospitals, HR managers and medical directors of all hospitals in the sample employed physicians from abroad in order to fill their vacancies. Rural hospitals did not see any alternative and regarded this undertaking as the only way to maintain the functionality of their hospitals, as expressed by one of the medical directors:

It is essential for the functionality of our hospital as a regional health care provider that we employ foreign physicians. Without that we can't do it (IP11: 59).[40]

38 „Das war super gut. Die waren äh, auch da wieder supermotiviert, engagiert und auch deutschtechnisch sehr, sehr gut strukturiert unterwegs (…) [U]nd ich habe jetzt aktuell letzte Woche, ähm, zwei, die in [dem anderen Krankenhaus, in dem ich tätig bin] ihr Praktikum gemacht haben, die würden gerne hier ihre Facharztausbildung absolvieren. Also den Kanal machen wir auch jetzt zurzeit, beackern wir ganz stark um da auch äh, da noch junge Hochschulabsolventen aus dem Ausland zu akquirieren" (IP31: 13).
39 „[W]ir müssen den Laden hier am Laufen halten" (IP06: 87).
40 „[E]s ist für die Funktionsfähigkeit unseres Krankenhauses als regionaler Gesundheitsversorger unerlässlich, dass wir ausländische Ärzte beschäftigen. Ohne das, können wir's nicht" (IP11: 59).

CEE migrant physicians were employed in German hospitals at the same conditions as German (-trained) physicians. They were meant to fill official positions provided in the hospitals including all duties and benefits (e.g. IP06: 121; IP22: 123).

When asked for the criteria applied to the employment of migrant physicians, the respondents based their answers on previous experiences they had and challenges they met in this respect. Their accounts included bureaucratic, cultural, linguistic, as well as professional aspects and strongly stressed the demand-driven character of this undertaking.

5.3.1 Bureaucratic implications

The interviewees described their staff shortages as occasionally being so severe that vacancies had to be filled immediately in order to guarantee full patient care. Therefore, employment had to be gapless, and had to occur fast. Bureaucratic procedures delaying the process were hence regarded as an additional burden hampering smooth hospital operations.

Although the bureaucratic process for migrant physicians from EU countries to practice medicine in Germany has been tremendously facilitated, application for the medical license and its issuance still requires up to six weeks. Documents and application forms are submitted and evaluated for equivalency, language certificates proofed, and in some Laender German proficiency with regard to medical, technical terms must pass additional oral tests conducted by the respective medical association. In contrast, German (-trained) doctors received their medical license with their final exam at medical school. Consequently, they could take up employment immediately, as one of the interviewees elucidated:

We're happy about every German application, which we receive, that is for sure (…). In the end when I've a German applicant, when someone has finished their medical studies, they've their medical license and can start to work here tomorrow. When we've a foreign applicant we've to go through all these formalities. That takes about five, normally four to six weeks (IP13: 181-185).[41]

---

41 „Also wir freuen uns über jede deutsche Bewerbung, die kommt, das ist klar. (…) Letztendlich, wenn ich
'nen deutschen Bewerber habe, wenn jemand mit dem Medizinstudium fertig ist, der hat seine Approbation,
der kann morgen anfangen, hier zu arbeiten. Ehm, wenn wir jetzt einen ausländischen Bewerber haben,
dann müssen wir auch diese ganzen Formalitäten machen, das dauert dann so fünf, vier bis sechs Wochen in
der Regel. Wenn alles vorhanden ist, es sei denn, es müssen noch Dokumente nachgereicht werden. Und
schon alleine dieses ganze Prozedere, ne?" (IP13: 181-185).

The account shows the recruitment of German (-trained) physicians to be preferable, underlining the reluctance of HR managers towards the recruitment from abroad. The period when migrant physicians were deemed fit for service could be additionally delayed if they had already completed residency abroad, and aimed to have their training formally recognised in Germany to be able to practice as medical specialist in their field. To that end, physicians received a certificate of conformity in their home countries stating that the respective qualifications meet EU standards. However, the responsibilities of medical specialists in the same discipline and the content of their training could differ across countries (IP06: 38). The bureaucratic procedures following from such a case were very long and thus did not meet the often ad hoc-demand of the hospitals, as illustrated by one of the HR managers:

If you need a physician for the department of gynaecology then you need them for this field. Then it doesn't help if the [responsible] district government tells you "OK, you've selected this physician, but they've to complete a structured period of adjustment. Six months internal medicine, six months surgery and only then they can work in gynaecology." That means I've got them one year here with us, not as a physician, but on the way to become one and can't employ them in gynaecology. That also means the vacancy still exists in that case and this doesn't help me at all (IP26: 70).[42]

Albeit the bureaucratic process of the recruitment of migrant physicians from CEE EU member states could occasionally be very time consuming, it can be expected that the recruitment of physicians from non-EU countries is even lengthier. Non-EU doctors aiming to practice medicine in Germany required both a residence and work permit before they can apply for a professional permit for which eligibility is checked individually (see ch. 2.2.3). It appears that by recruiting CEE migrant doctors from EU member countries, the HR managers intended to circumvent these bureaucratic procedures. Due to the freedom of movement of EU citizens, and the EU directive 2005/36/EC on harmonisation of professional qualifications, their qualifications were accepted without further ado. However, the EU membership of the physicians' home countries was mentioned only rarely by the respondents when justifying why they recruited mainly CEE doctors (IP26: 70; IP31: 8).

---

42 „[W]enn Sie zum Beispiel eine Ärztin oder einen Arzt für den Fachbereich Gynäkologie brauchen, dann brauchen Sie den für diesen Fachbereich. Da hilft es ihnen nicht, wenn die [zuständige] Bezirksregierung (…) Ihnen sagt, "OK, Sie haben sich jetzt diesen Arzt ausgesucht, aber der muss jetzt erst eine strukturierte Anpassungszeit machen. Sechs Monate Innere, sechs Monate Chirurgie und erst dann darf er in die Gynäkologie gehen." Das heißt ich habe den ein Jahr bei uns, nicht als Arzt, aber auf dem Weg zum Arzt, und kann ihn nicht in der Gynäkologie einsetzen. Das heißt also die Stellenvakanz bleibt mir an der Stelle und da ist mir nicht wirklich geholfen" (IP26: 70).

5.3.2 Cultural implications

When queried about employing migrant physicians from CEE countries, HR managers and medical directors stressed an alleged cultural proximity in terms of mentality, common values, and attitude to work of these physicians. Interestingly, while the subjects constituting the boundaries were the same, the definition of in- and out-groups differed. In any case, cultural proximity was highly appreciated for ensuring a frictionless daily routine on ward.

Stressing the similar mentality of the physicians, recruited from Hungary, Romania and the Baltic countries, the HR managers emphasised how well they blend in with the other hospital staff on-site: "The kind of people, I put this in quotes, actually go well with the house. In terms of comprehension and integration the people I could recruit are very easy to integrate" (IP31: 8).[43] This notion was not only formed based on a comparison with German (-trained) physicians, but also in contrast to migrant physicians who did not match the interviewees' expectations. Almost all respondents who discussed this issue drew comparisons between CEE migrant physicians on the one hand, and other groups of migrant physicians on the other. Interviewees referred to a different understanding of medicine and different values, for example regarding medical care for the elderly (IP26: 32), and contact with women. The latter was a topic that many interviewees mentioned and were concerned about with regard to the interaction of the respective medical doctors with female colleagues, nurses, and patients treating them with a lack of respect and not being willing to accept a woman as their superior (e.g. IP13: 227; IP22: 93; IP31: 21). While the content of perceived cultural clashes remained similar, the boundaries that were made ranged from mainly out-grouping medical doctors from Arabic and African countries, to a less often out-grouping of those from Bulgaria and Romania, as stated by an interviewee representing a rural hospital:

If you go further with Bulgaria and Romania, especially Romania. (...) In Romania there's a little different approach. Especially maybe in special hospital perceptions. When I look at gynaecology/obstetrics and you have a Romanian physician, masculin – complicated. The image is a different one, isn't it? And ... let me use this as an example, your boyfriend maybe cooks and serves you the food. That would not be happening there (IP06: 22).[44]

---

43 „[D]er Menschenschlag sage ich mal in Anführungszeichen, passt eigentlich sehr gut zum Haus. Also die Leute, die ich da rekrutieren konnte, die sind vom Verständnis her, von der Integration her sehr, sehr gut einbindbar" (IP31: 8).

44 „Wenn man weitergeht mit Bulgarien und Rumänien. Vor allen Dingen Rumänien. (...) [I]n Rumänien ist das doch etwas anders von der Auffassung. Vor allen Dingen vielleicht in speziellen Klinikbildern. Wenn ich die Gyn/Geburtshilfe mir anschaue und Sie haben einen rumänischen Arzt, also maskulin - kompliziert. Ne, weil das Bild ist ein anderes, ne? Und der... hier sag ich mal, Ihr Freund kocht vielleicht, ne und tut Sie bedienen und das würde dort nicht stattfinden können" (IP06: 22).

Here the boundary was drawn narrower excluding doctors from the most recently accessed EU member countries ascribing to them the same traditional ideas of gender roles that were also attested to male physicians from African and Arab countries. Religious values also played a role. HR managers and medical directors justified their reluctance to employ physicians from countries with Muslim background for example with their concern about the comfort and well-being of the patients.

Well, that's simply the perception of the human being. Can we as humans help an injured person? Or is the other person so heavily injured that we've to give them in other hands. I mean Allah's hands. Yes. And I believe there is a different way of thinking, too (IP26: 32).[45]

In the same vein, some of those representing church-sponsored hospitals emphasised the necessary match of the candidate with the mission statement of their facility, particularly the Christian values they represent (IP06: 18; IP26: 14). In general, the HR managers and medical directors insisted on the necessity that migrant physicians adapted to the local work culture (e.g. IP11: 49).

5.3.3 Linguistic implications

German language proficiency was stressed as the most crucial and essential criterion in the recruitment of migrant physicians by the HR managers and medical directors (e.g. IP11: 27; IP12: 8; IP22: 22). They emphasised the importance of sound German language skills for smooth hospital operations in different respects. Firstly, they regarded German language skills as crucial for the physicians' integration in terms of a cultural adaptation, and secondly due to the interactive character of the medical profession. In light of these standards, they concluded that the B2 certificate is neither sufficient nor indicative of actual language skills. Moreover, there is heavy criticism lodged at migrant physicians who communicate in their native language among compatriots, which is perceived as means of undesirable boundary making between the migrant physicians on the one, and the German speaking hospital staff on the other hand (IP26: 93). In this respect, respondents also emphasised the need to master the German language, since German proficiency would promote not only the cultural integration of the migrant doctors, but also the acceptance and recognition on the part of colleagues, other hospital staff and patients, as one

---

45 „Ja, also da ist einfach der Blick auf den Menschen, ne. Können wir als, als Menschen selber einem verletzten Menschen helfen? Oder ist der Mensch so schwer verletzt, dass wir äh, ihn in andere Hände legen. Sprich in Allahs Hände. Ja. Und ich glaube da gibt es auch noch einen unterschiedlichen Denkprozess" (IP26: 32).

of the respondents emphasised: "The more they know the language, the better the integration, comprehension and acceptance" (IP06: 76)[46]. With regard to the patient-doctor relationship, understanding was not only regarded as crucial in an intercultural sense, but also with respect to the recognition of the migrant physicians in their capacity as medical doctors on the part of the patients due the profession's interactive character, as one medical director stated, physicians "work with humans not with machines" (IP16: 44)[47]. Patients tended to interpret incorrect and insecure ways of expressing oneself as incompetence and concluded a lack of professional qualification (IP27: 58). In this respect, German language proficiency was also seen as crucial for confident self-presentation when interacting with patients:

It's always a question of how self-confident a physician presents themselves. (…) You can only be truly self-confident when you speak the language, so you can communicate well. It's always about the language. You may be professionally qualified, but when the patient can't communicate with you, then we've a problem (IP16: 60-62).[48]

As the account above demonstrates, patients feel uncomfortable and insecure with migrant physicians because they appear unable to understand the patients on the one hand, and to express themselves in a way that is understandable for patients, on the other (IP15: 51; IP13: 175). This was stated to apply especially to older patients or those limited in their faculty of hearing and expressing themselves. Consequently, deficient language skills and listening comprehension would cause discomfort as well as anger on the part of patients (IP26: 16; IP16: 56). The ability to appease and comfort patients was seen as crucial for medical doctors: "A doctor's personal care about a patient is the bottom line. Sometimes you can cure someone just with care. And if that is impossible because of the language basis or barrier, then there are problems" (IP16: 44).[49]

Apart from interactions with patients, also those with nurses, medical colleagues and bureaucratic affairs were mentioned to emphasise the indispensability of German language skills for migrant physicians in German hospitals. Hence, the lack thereof was said to occasionally cause displeasure among other hospital staff, for example when migrant physicians were overwhelmed with

---

46 „Je besser die die Sprache können, desto besser ist die Integration und das Verständnis und die Akzeptanz" (IP06: 76).

47 „(…) arbeiten mit Menschen und nicht mit Geräten" (IP16: 44).

48 „[E]s kommt natürlich immer darauf an, wie ein Arzt, eine Ärztin sich gibt, wie selbstbewusst sie auftreten. (…) [R]ichtig selbstbewusst kann man nur auftreten wenn man auch der Sprache mächtig ist, dass man sich auch richtig unterhalten kann. Das ist, dreht sich sehr, sehr viel um die Sprache. Da kannst Du fachlich noch so qualifiziert sein, wenn das da dran hapert, dass der Patient sich mit einem nicht unterhalten kann, dann haben wir ein Problem" (IP16: 60-62).

49 „[D]ie persönliche Zuwendung eines Arztes an einen Patienten [ist] das alles Entscheidende. Man kann manchmal nur mit Zuwendung jemanden gesund machen. Und wenn das wegen der sprachlichen Basis oder Barriere nicht geht, dann gibt's Probleme" (IP16:44).

bureaucratic tasks such as writing discharge letters and had to rely on administrative staff to help them (IP13: 85), or when language issues occurred repeatedly and caused impatience and stress for everyone involved (IP06:91). Dissatisfaction about the hampered daily routine and cooperation on the ward were said to particularly affect the relationship between migrant physicians and the nurses. Apart from complications during work procedures, nurses would like patients interpret migrant physicians' difficulties in communicating in German as a sign of incompetence, and consequently, a lack of authority. This amplified the already tense relationship that was said to often exist between young junior doctors who had just started residency, but were authorised to give instructions, and the more experienced nurses tasked to carry them out:

Partly they need a reasonable structure, that's clear and they take a critical look at it, when the processes don't run smoothly. (…) And then such a status as a foreigner who, let's say, can't yet act self-confidently, but still is in the role to give instructions and has to have a certain authority. And as mentioned, they can't adequately fulfil this role (IP27: 64).[50]

Thus, this experience-based advantage was conceived as reversing the usual hierarchical order leading to occasional conflicts.

In sum, HR managers and medical directors concluded that the B2-certificate required by the medical associations for obtaining the medical license was insufficient for practicing such an interactive profession (e.g. IP22: 33; IP27: 30). Furthermore, they stated that it did not inform about the actual language skills of the migrant physicians (e.g. IP11: 29; 15: 34), and asserted to assess the migrant doctors' language competence themselves, either during a first contact on the phone (IP22: 33), or during the job interview on-site (IP31: 10). One HR manager stated that he would prefer to employ migrant physicians with more elaborate German skills, such as in the case of candidates who had already completed their studies at a German university, thus also being familiar with technical terms in German (IP26: 16).

Almost all of the interviewees agreed on language proficiency as the most crucial skill required from migrant physicians. Additionally, respondents representing city hospitals declared to not employ migrant doctors with insufficient German proficiency. However, one medical director argued that initially weak language skills were likely to be quickly improved once the physician was working on-site.

---

50 „Zum Teil brauchen sie [das Pflegepersonal] eine vernünftige Anordnung, is-, ist ja klar, und sehen das dann sehr kritisch, wenn das dann nicht so glatt läuft. (…) Ähm, macht sich dann so ein, ein Status als Ausländer, der da noch nicht so, sagen wir mal so, selbstbewusst auftreten kann, aber trotzdem eine Anordnungskompetenz hat und auch eine gewisse Autorität ja haben muss. Äh, die kann er nicht so, wie sagt man, zur Verfügung stellen, ja" (IP27: 64).

If we then have to face that, OK, with the language it doesn't work that well yet, but they're intelligent and, let me put it that way, willing to work @(.)@,[51] interested, hardworking, then you can assume that they're going to learn German as well. And from experience I can say that they learn quickly. Therefore, you don't have to raise the expectations too high concerning the language. They can learn that within half a year quite well, can't they? (IP27: 30)[52]

High expectations regarding migrant physicians' language skills could not always be adhered in pressing situations of staff shortages. This reveals that even without German language proficiency, a professional induction of migrant physicians is possible. Nevertheless, while most of the HR managers and medical directors stuck to their rather reluctant attitude stressing high demands, this latter respondent was the only one to show a more open and supportive attitude towards the recruitment of migrant physicians.

5.3.4 Professional implications

With respect to professional criteria, the expectations of HR managers and medical directors towards migrant physicians were rather basic in terms of fulfilling the formal requirements for suitability. However, they regarded previously gained practical experiences in a German hospital as beneficial for smooth hospital operations.

While German language proficiency was a recruitment criterion that was applied to both junior physicians and medical specialists, professional skills and knowledge were expected to a higher degree from the latter than from the former. As the former just graduated from medical school, no clinical experience was expected (IP11: 27), while medical specialists had to master the respective treatments and therapies of their medical field. Based on the harmonisation of professional training across the EU member countries, the respective professional qualifications of the CEE migrant physicians were mutually recognised, and were in general also evaluated as equal to the one of German (-trained) doctors by the interviewees (e.g. IP06: 72, IP15: 52, IP27: 50).

Moreover, medical specialists were especially welcome if having completed residency in a German hospital, since they were already familiar with the procedures on-site:

---

51 The "@" indicates that the interviewee laughed while speaking. This applies throughout all interview quotations. For further information see attachment iv.

52 „[W]enn wir dann sehen, OK, sprachlich geht das so eigentlich noch nicht richtig, aber äh, ein, ein, das ist ein intelligenter Mensch und äh, ich sag jetzt mal, arbeitswillig @(.)@, interessiert, fleißig, dann kann man ja davon ausgehen, dass er das Deutsch auch lernt. Und die Erfahrung die ist auch so, dass die das dann schnell lernen. Deswegen muss man da nicht unbedingt die, äh, die Ansprüche zu hoch stellen was die Sprache angeht. Das können die innerhalb von einem halben Jahr ganz gut lernen, ne" (IP27: 30).

As mentioned, one big plus, for example, we've Syrians now who for example have completed their specialist training in Germany, then went back to Syria and now returned to Germany. Not a problem at all, don't you think? Works very well and we're now checking whether we can recruit someone else as well (IP11: 53).[53]

This was perceived as particularly beneficial, since differing professional orders between the medical profession in Germany and the ones in the physicians' countries of study, again hampered smooth working procedures. Hence, practical shares during medical studies were understood to be more extensive in Germany than in some of the migrant doctors' countries of studies (IP22: 35/37). Accordingly, they would bring less practical experience, and consequently need more time of training until they would be able to independently take over responsibilities. At the same time, the insistence of using local standards implies an attempt to protect local ways of conduct against influences and alterations by others.

Nevertheless, in spite of these expectations towards migrant physicians, in the end HR managers and medical directors admitted that in very pressing situations they were not in the position to request too much, but were forced to proceed rather randomly in their recruitment – something that applied to both hospitals located in remote, as well as urban areas: "[Some] departments have 2-3 open positions and therefore are very pleased about everybody. That means that they don't recruit according to quality criteria, but hire whoever is applying" (IP15: 36).[54]

To summarize, HR managers' and medical directors' demands towards migrant physicians suggest they prefer them to be trained in Germany, because they expect these physicians to be similar to German physicians and well-adjusted to German professional culture. This corresponds to the reluctant attitude that the respondents conveyed when complaining of a lack of action taken on the part of the government to address the increasing demand of medical doctors in Germany. The boundary making with regard to non-EU physicians supports this search of likeness and implies a hierarchy among the migrant physicians in terms of desirability. Given that HR managers and medical directors hired migrant physicians who did not fulfil these expectations stresses the demand-driven and ad-hoc character of the recruitment.

---

53 „[D]as ist ein großes Plus z.B., wie gesagt, wir haben Syrer jetzt z.B. die in Deutschland ihre Facharztweiterbildung gemacht haben, dann nach Syrien zurückgegangen sind, jetzt wiedergekommen sind. Überhaupt kein Problem, ja? Funktioniert super gut und, und wir gucken jetzt gerade, dass wir noch jemanden rekrutieren" (IP11: 53).

54 „[Manche] Abteilungen haben 2-3 Stellen nicht besetzt und sind natürlich für jeden dankbar. Das wird also dann nicht so unbedingt nach Qualitätsmerkmalen gemacht, sondern da wird einfach genommen, wer sich gerade bewirbt" (IP15: 36).

5.4 "Then they see how it works, don't they?"[55]

In order to help the migrant doctors to get settled, some of the hospitals provided incorporation measures during the physicians' initial phase on-site as summarised in table 5.[56]

Table 5 Measures of incorporation taken by the hospitals

		Hospitals						
		Urban			Rural			
		C	D	E	A	B	F	G
Incorporation Measures								
Practical support	bureaucracy					x	x	x
	financial support				x	(x)*		x
	flat hunting		x		x	x		x
	accommodation upon arrival				x	x	x	x
Linguistic incorporation	in-house German class					x	x	
	external German class			(x)		(x)		x
Professional incorporation	work shadowing					x		x
	mentoring		x	x	x	x		x
	batch card					x		

* () = not as a rule

Source: Own table

Since the representatives of the city hospitals did not engage in active recruitment of migrant physicians, they also did not offer incorporation measures. Thus, there is a clear distinction between the different facilities related to their respective degrees of physician shortages. All hospitals besides city hospitals, offered different incorporation measures, ranging from practical support upon arrival to professional and linguistic support.

---

55 „[D]ann sehen die ja wie das läuft, ne?" (IP06: 66).
56 Since the table is based on the qualitative interview material and not a systematic survey with closed questions the provided information might be incomplete.

5.4.1 Practical support upon arrival

The incorporation measures provided by hospitals began with supporting the migrant physicians with practical matters to get set up on-site. These included bureaucratic tasks with regard to the issuance of the medical license, the employment of the migrant doctor in the hospital, as well as non-work related aspects, such as finding a place to live. The effort was not only made to guarantee a fast start of work, but also to ensure the physicians' comfort with the intention to bind them to the hospital in the long term.

A number of bureaucratic tasks had to be completed upon the migrant physicians' arrival including application for the medical license. Since these formalities tended to be very complex (particularly for non-native speakers), the minimum help that was offered in most facilities was bureaucratic support. Due to a close contact to the local authorities particularly in smaller towns, procedures such as applying for the medical license could be quickly dealt with by the respective human resource departments (e.g. IP11: 35; IP13: 93; IP26: 22). In some cases, bureaucratic tasks were taken care of by recruitment agencies with which the HR managers cooperated. In other cases, one respondent stated he would make sure to even accompany migrant physicians to official appointments with authorities himself:

[It is important to me that] they've an absolute contact person who guides them. I always say in the employment process if this doesn't work they should address us, so we can jump in. Yes, this is primarily in our interest, too. And actually works excellently (IP31: 29).[57]

Apart from these professional matters, some hospitals also assisted the migrant physicians with bureaucratic tasks that were not directly related to their employment, but were needed in order to get settled. This included practical issues such as opening a bank account, finding health insurance and so on. While in most cases the respective human resource department took care of this, in one hospital each migrant physician was assigned a mentor (IP11: 33; IP13: 31). During the time CEE migrant physicians had to wait to receive their medical license (approximately up to six weeks), most of the facilities invited them for work shadowing on-site. Since the migrant doctors were not fully employed during that time, they did not receive full payment, but were – in a few cases – provided with a kind of pocket money of about 500€ (IP06: 54). Moreover, some of the hospitals provided board and accommodation during that time. The kind of accommodation that was offered differed. While some facilities were

---

57   „[Mir ist wichtig, d]ass sie einen absoluten Ansprechpartner haben und auch eine Begleitung erfahren.
      Wenn nicht, sage ich ihnen auch immer in der, in der Einstellung, sollen sie sich bitte vertrauensvoll an uns
      wenden, dann werden wir es dann machen. Ja. Ist ja auch in erster Linie in unserem Interesse. Und das
      funktioniert eigentlich hervorragend" (IP31: 29).

able to provide apartments in the hospital area (IP26: 20; IP31: 87), others provided hotel rooms. The hotel rooms were either entirely (IP06: 87) or at least partially paid for by the hospitals (IP13: 31), and the apartments were available at a reduced rate. As the apartments on the hospital area provided by some facilities were un-furnished, one of them offered the physicians to choose furniture from IKEA online, which was then bought and assembled prior to the physicians' arrival so that they had at least a bed (IP31: 165). The migrant physicians had the opportunity to stay in these apartments after taking up full employment, and only then had to pay the full price.

Hospitals also provided assistance with finding an apartment. This is one of the few offers that also an interviewee representing one of the city hospitals mentioned. Nonetheless, this support was not specifically targeted at migrant physicians, but provided for all doctors moving to the hospital's location when taking up employment there (IP22: 55). In the case of small, remotely located hospitals, this reflects the facilities' need to attract medical doctors from abroad. While a city hospital only supports the apartment search, one of the rural hospitals even covers the costs for the rent before the medical license was issued and the work contract was signed (IP06: 58). The same hospital also helped with finding furniture if needed.

The intended function of these measures was not only to attract migrant physicians, but to also keep them on-site. HR managers of rurally located hospitals were explicitly endeavoured to also establish family members who possibly accompanied the migrant physician by making sure to find them a nice apartment (IP31: 87), to assist the partner with the job search, and to find a place in a local child care facility if needed (IP06: 106). Thus, in particular respondents from rural hospitals aimed to ensure a long term employment of the respective migrant doctor in the hospital:

We want to integrate them. Otherwise it doesn't pay off. The children don't have any problem, in kindergarten, school – they're rather ahead. But if the partner with the language maybe, or has a job... (…) Normally, they shouldn't remain tourists, should they? But integrate themselves, don't you think? We want a long lasting connection, that they establish themselves (IP06: 30-32).[58]

Fear of potentially losing migrant physicians again was particularly articulated on the part of respondents of remotely located hospitals. Interviewees stressed the wish for migrant physicians to stay in the respective hospital on a long-term basis, as well as the disappointment on the part of colleagues and other hospital staff that had made an effort to welcome and incorporate the respective migrant physician on-site (IP06: 93). Additionally, that would mean a great

---

58   „Wir wollen die integrieren, die Leute. Sonst trägt das nicht aus. Die Kinder haben kein Problem, ne. Kindergarten, Schule - die sind eher on top. Aber wenn der Partner mit der Sprache vielleicht oder ein Beruf hat... (…) [D]as sollen also in der Regel keine Touris bleiben, ne? Sondern sich bei uns integrieren, ne? Wir wollen lange Verbindungen, dass die sich bei uns etablieren" (IP06: 30-32).

loss, given the money and time invested into their incorporation: "We invest a lot of money and hard work to train the people and then they leave, that would be fatal. Yes. Happens again and again. Can't be completely prevented, I assume" (IP31: 131).[59] The main cause for this concern on the part of representatives of the rural hospitals was the remote location of small towns with limited free time activities and entertainment on offer. Interviewees were worried that the migrant physicians got socially isolated and felt lonely: "Another big problem is when physicians come here, they lack contact to others. Here that's, well, we're just a small town" (IP13: 95).[60] In particular, since many of the migrant physicians were of young age, interviewees had the impression that some of them missed home and would spend their free time mainly using the internet to stay in touch with friends and family at home, instead of socialising on-site (IP06: 85).

5.4.2 Linguistic incorporation

As illustrated above, HR managers and medical directors identified German language proficiency as the most crucial criterion for migrant doctors to be successful in a German hospital. Accordingly, the provision of linguistic incorporation measures was a prominent topic. However, in spite of the consensus between most of the interviewees regarding the significance of sound German skills when practicing medicine in a German hospital, the responses to the question whether or not to provide a language class varied. Only one HR manager of a rural hospital viewed the hospital as being primarily responsible for their physicians' German language skills, and did not understand why in other facilities this was not taken care of:

I read some of the press articles saying "the share of foreigners [among physicians] is increasing", that's how it is, I can only confirm that. And where many…, or I think that's a problem of the hospitals that don't prioritise German, ensure that courses are offered (IP31: 57).[61]

In his hospital, work shadowing (provided by almost all facilities in the sample), was regarded as a first opportunity for migrant physicians to become familiar with the German language. Therefore, work shadowing was a requirement for all migrant physicians on-site. During that time, the hospital offered an intensive language class for the migrant physicians at a close-by language

---

59 „(…) [W]ir investieren viel Geld und Schweißblut die Leute auszubilden, dann gehen sie weg, das wäre natürlich fatal. Ja. Erlebt man immer wieder. Kann man ja wahrscheinlich nicht ganz unterbinden" (IP31: 131).

60 „Was auch ein großes Problem ist, wenn die Ärzte hierher kommen, sie haben kaum Anschluss. Das ist hier, wir sind nun mal ´ne Kleinstadt" (IP13: 95).

61 „[M]anche Presseartikel bekomme ich ja auch mit wo es heißt "der Ausländeranteil wächst", das ist so, kann ich nur bestätigen. Und wo viele, oder ich denke das ist ein Problem der Kliniken, äh, nicht dann dafür Sorge tragen, dass auch Deutsch da ganz klar vorne ansteht, wo dann auch Kurse angeboten werden" (IP31: 57).

school. Thus, the interviewee felt that the time the physicians spent waiting for the license was to be ideally used for German-language and work-life acculturation to prepare for work in the local hospital (IP31: 37). The class continued on after the migrant doctors had officially taken up employment, but took place off the job in order to make sure that the physicians were present and available on ward during their work time: "Everything takes place after work, otherwise the head physician is angry with me" (ibid).[62] Hence, there is a conflict of interests between the linguistic incorporation of the migrant physicians on the one, and the necessity for them to help out on ward on the other hand. In any case, no work time was granted to the physicians to improve their language skills. In order to reduce the timely effort, some hospital administrations offered German classes within the hospital building after official hours. In the smallest of the hospitals, classes were even demand-tailored and took place individually in a one-to-one setting (IP06: 62/64).

In the city hospitals, on the contrary, language learning was primarily regarded as the responsibility of the medical doctors themselves: "The training isn't only served on a tray, on a silver one, it's also about a certain own dedication in terms of learning the language. To me this is about self-commitment".[63] In line with their inactivity in terms of targeted recruitment from abroad, they did not offer language classes for migrant physicians. This might be due to the fact that they did not see the necessity, as they still had sufficient German (-trained) physicians to rely on. Additionally, they were likely to receive more applications for open positions than other hospitals. Thus, they could probably be more selective with regard to migrant physicians' language proficiency than other hospitals, and were not in need to deal with that matter. In contrast to representatives of rural hospitals, HR managers and medical directors of city hospitals still perceived their hospitals on the supply- rather than the demand-side of the market. In this position, they requested migrant physicians wanting to complete residency in their hospitals to fulfil this criterion of German proficiency. HR managers of remotely located hospitals shared that view, but could not always afford it. In situations when no physicians with sound German language skills were available, doctors with lower levels of German proficiency were employed. In order to address the deficiency, language classes were then offered, even if only under duress:

No. We offer that in individual cases, that we say "Ok, we contribute to the language courses", but that's not a rule. We admit that we do have a shortage of qualified persons,

---

62 „[D]as läuft alles außerhalb der Arbeitszeit, sonst springt mir ja der Chefarzt auch wieder an den Hals" (ibid).
63 „[D]ie Ausbildung wird ja nur nicht auf dem Tablett serviert auf einem silbernen, da gehört auch ein gewisses eigenes Engagement, was, was, äh, das Lernen der Sprache angeht, das gehört für mich, läuft für mich unter Eigenengagement" (IP16: 120).

but not such a severe need that on principal we finance preparatory courses or similar things (IP11: 31).[64]

In this hospital, migrant physicians were asked to later reimburse the costs initially covered by the facility. They did not only ask for motivational but also financial commitment.

Motivational commitment was something that many interviewees claimed to miss. They complained that migrant physicians would not show enough initiative on their own, would not sufficiently appreciate the provided language class, and perceive it as additional burden rather than as an opportunity (IP26: 20). One respondent identified the reason for this perceived lack of commitment in the current market situation. He implied that the migrant physicians would take advantage of the fact that they were urgently needed:

Those who came in 2004 and 2003, they back then took private lessons. They saw that, "I've to speak the language and then it works." But the interest is maybe declining, of course because the people know through online and other media, "We're a scarce and demanded good. I don't necessarily have to do that. They should make an effort" (IP06: 76).[65]

Another interviewee suggested a different reason for why migrant physicians might be reluctant to take part in the provided language course. His first assumption was that the classes were too heterogeneous in terms of the language levels of the participants – which cannot apply to the one-to-one class offered by one of the facilities in the sample. His second notion was that migrant doctors might perceive the German class as little helpful for their daily routine, and would better pick up the language learning-by-doing, as he elucidated:

I believe it's almost better they learn the language in their daily routine. That's probably the general experience. But, if I look at it from a different perspective, if a German goes to America, even if they know more or less English from school, nevertheless they really learn the language when they're in a family and have to communicate every day. Then after four weeks you know how they speak, don't you? *(IP27: 44)[66]*

---

64 „Nein. Wir machen das in Einzelfällen, dass wir, dass wir sagen "Ok, wir beteiligen uns an Sprachkursen", aber das ist nicht die Regel. Wir haben schon Fachkräftemangel, das muss man schon sagen, aber nicht so bittere Not, dass wir, eh dass wir grundsätzlich Vorbereitungskurse finanzieren oder ähnliche Dinge" (IP11: 31).

65 „[D]ie, die 2004 und 2003 zu uns gekommen sind, da haben die Privatunterricht genommen. Die haben das gesehen, ,Ich muss die Sprache können und dann läuft das.' Aber, das Interesse nimmt vielleicht auch so ein bisschen ab, weil natürlich die Leute über das Internet und andere Medien wissen, ,Wir sind ja 'ne Mangelware, wir sind ja begehrt. Das muss ich vielleicht gar nicht unbedingt machen. Sollen die sich mal drehen'" (IP06: 76).

66 „[I]ch meine es ist fast besser die lernen es hier einfach im täglichen Umgang. Wahrscheinlich ist das überhaupt äh, auch sonst die Erfahrung. Also, äh, wenn ich mal was anderes sehe, wenn ein Deutscher nach Amerika geht, die können zwar alle aus der Schule ein bisschen, mehr oder weniger Englisch. So richtig lernen tun sie es einfach wenn sie dann in einer Familie sind und jeden Tag mitreden müssen, dann weiß man nach vier Wochen wie, wie die reden, ja" (IP27: 44).

Hence, he doubted the usefulness and effectiveness of language classes in general for the migrant physicians' acquisition of the needed language skills, thus taking a very different view compared to the other respondents.

5.4.3 Professional Incorporation

Apart from assisting migrant physicians with getting settled, some hospitals also offered measures to professionally incorporate them in the daily routine. In most cases, however, these were not specifically targeted at migrant physicians, but were provided for all doctors who were new on-site.

Most hospitals invited the migrant physicians for work shadowing during the time they spent waiting for their medical license, which usually took up to six weeks. During this period, physicians were not allowed to practice independently as they were not officially employed yet. However, they got the chance to follow fellow physicians around on ward to see what the procedures on-site were like and to become familiar with the new work environment. In one hospital, this orientation phase was additionally organised by using a batch card system. Physicians took these batch cards to different departments within the hospital where they met the responsible colleagues who explained certain procedures and the handling of certain technical equipment. Thus, they collected signatures on their batch card until all indicated stages were ticked off (IP11: 33). This incorporation measure was not specifically targeted at migrant physicians, but also applied to German (-trained) medical doctors who were new in the respective hospital.

Once physicians had received their medical license and taken up employment, they were allowed to practice medicine and usually started treating patients immediately. However, especially junior physicians in residency were initially supervised by experienced colleagues. This mentoring arrangement in which senior physicians were assigned as mentors to young junior physicians, was applied to both migrant and German (-trained) physicians in most of the hospitals in the sample, and was also mentioned by two representatives of city hospitals (e.g. IP06: 56; IP11: 33; IP13: 31; IP22: 55). However, again this measure was common to incorporate not only migrant physicians, but also German (-trained) beginners. All junior doctors in residency had one main contact person whom to address with questions and concerns regarding their specialist training, and who they met up with to discuss their current situation on a frequent basis. Apart from that, other colleagues were said to be approachable with urgent and ad-hoc questions. Accordingly, one interviewee explained that all beginners in his hospital started out on the ward for inpatient admission because there was a prevalence of doctors and therefore, always somebody to approach in cases of insecurity. Moreover, that was where young physicians learned all basic measures (IP27: 46). Besides help from colleagues, all physicians received introductory information at an event set up for all new employees of the hospital, and had the opportunity to participate in external trainings as part of their residency (IP16: 30; IP31: 43).

Apart from this rather general information on the one hand, and information that was specific for certain medical fields on the other, no information or incorporation measure was mentioned that was targeted particularly at physicians who were professionally socialised in a different medical system. Also, none of these measures were tailored specifically to the needs of non-German (-trained) physicians who did not already gain work experience during an internship in a German hospital, who did not grow up with the German health care system, or who did not learn about how it operates at university. Since most of the migrant physicians in the sample started in the German hospital as junior physicians in residency, they were treated just like German (-trained) beginners. The only factor that was identified to hamper this procedure, while simultaneously emphasizing the crucial difference between German (-trained) and migrant physicians, was the level of German proficiency in the latter. One of the medical directors remarked:

Someone who already speaks very good German will be treated like a normal new assistant who has just graduated from a German university, meaning they speak German and are incorporated. Someone who doesn't speak German too well yet, of course you can't confront them with patients in that way. That means they need much more guidance. Of course that's time consuming (…). Well, to be clear about it, they've always an assistant by hand, someone they follow and who shows them everything and trains them (IP16: 22-24).[67]

Thus, language problems gave occasion for the provision of additional assistance. At the same time, the description of such help as 'time intensive' implies that the need for its provision was perceived as a burden. This confirms the assumption stated above that HR managers and medical directors' primary interest was the fast and easy integration of migrant physicians into the daily routine of the hospital. Given the pressing shortage of physicians, the respondents argued that there was no time for extensive settling in, one interviewee explained: "The hospital business is running and you have to fill a gap. So you don't have time to say; now we start one-year training. That's not very likely to happen" (IP06: 66).[68] Hence, instead of providing professional incorporation

---

67 „Jemand der sehr gutes Deutsch schon spricht, der wird quasi wie ein normaler Frischassistent behandelt, der von einer deutschen Uni kommt, also deutschsprachig ist und eingearbeitet. Jemand der der deutschen Sprache nicht so mächtig ist, den können Sie natürlich nicht so auf Patienten loslassen. Das heißt, der braucht wesentlich mehr Begleitung. Das ist natürlich zeitintensiv dann. (…) Äh, so ganz platt ausgedrückt, der hat immer einen Assi an der Hand, ähm mit dem er erst einmal immer mitläuft und der ihm alles zeigt und ihn im wahrsten Sinne des Wortes anlernt" (IP16: 22-24).

68 „[D]as Geschäft läuft ja weiter und man tut ja eine Lücke besetzten. Da hat man schlecht Zeit zu sagen, jetzt machen wir einen einjährigen Einarbeitungslehrgang. Das wird eher nicht stattfinden" (IP06: 66).

measures to address potential barriers and problems in a demand-tailored way, migrant physicians were expected to immediately fill the vacancies they were employed for, fulfilling all responsibilities. Interviewees relied on the effect of learning-by-doing, as well as on migrant physicians who arrived in their hospitals earlier to take over this task (ibid.).

To summarize, the level of practical support given to migrant physicians upon arrival and incorporation measures demonstrates the demand-driven character of their recruitment. This is highlighted by high expectations mainly on the part of representatives of the city hospitals, and with respect to language also on the part of representatives of the rural hospitals. The measures are mainly ad-hoc in nature, thus aimed at quickly filling vacancies, but not interested in sustainable human resource development. Particularly linguistic incorporation measures were perceived as a burden that was blamed on physicians rather than institutional shortcomings. German proficiency is a requirement commonly expected from immigrants on the part of the German society, and is thus not limited to the medical sphere.

5.5 "That is not going to be a temporary solution"[69]

Evaluating the recruitment of CEE physicians, and reflecting upon future perspectives, HR managers and medical directors expressed ambivalence about the multicultural situation on ward, weighing up disadvantages and advantages. They agreed that the dependence of German hospitals would not stop in the near future, but would rather expand, also affecting the city hospitals to a larger degree.

Despite their general dissatisfaction with the situation, many respondents valued the recruitment of migrant physicians as enrichment. This notion was expressed in two different ways. One aspect HR managers and medical directors greatly appreciated about the CEE migrant physicians was the diligence and commitment with which they approached their work (IP31: 153). Compared to their young, German (-trained) counterparts, they were seen as more eager and motivated. Hence, they were regarded as having the potential for being role models to the German physicians on-site: "[B]ecause they work with a different diligence, (...) they can definitely be a role model for a younger German who thinks they can approach everything with a slower pace" (IP27: 103).[70] In contrast to the focus on a so called work-life-balance that the interviewees had identified as being prevalent among the German (-trained) junior

69 „[D]as wird keine Übergangslösung bleiben" (IP13: 179).
70 „[W]eil die mit einem anderen Fleiß herangehen, (...) können sie durchaus mal vorbildhaft sein für einen jüngeren Deutschen, der vielleicht meint das Ganze etwas gemütlicher angehen zu können" (IP27: 103).

physicians, they felt that the CEE migrant doctors were ready to make a bigger effort with respect to work (see also IP27: 93): "They are happy to be here and step on the gas. And they don't discuss long" (IP31: 111).[71] The migrant doctors' diverse language skills were evaluated as another relevant enrichment for the hospitals. Especially in hospitals close to the Polish border with a number of Polish patients, and in those with a high share of migrant patients this was perceived as very helpful (IP13: 175, IP22: 127, IP27: 99). In the same vein, one interviewee valued the cultural knowledge migrant physicians contributed when treating patients with the same national and religious background, respectively (IP 22: 127). Despite this positive outlook, he also mentioned the negative consequences:

That does help in the routine whereas it also slows down the routine, because you do something out of your own German way of thinking and that's completely different to a foreign or immigrated doctor. Of course this increases the effort to explain what's going on or fuels the misunderstanding if you don't communicate well (ibid.).[72]

The recruitment of migrant doctors was additionally treasured for its qualitative value of precious experiences of intercultural exchange (IP13: 175), and esteemed as elevating: "[B]ecause in the end it reduces prejudices, you broaden your horizon" (IP27: 99).[73] At the same time however, cultural differences were perceived as threatening:

Well, I can only appreciate that, can't I? If cultures grow together then there's also an understanding of cultures, every culture has to tolerate the other. This should never be a one-sided business and overrun. To me, that's very, very important (IP26: 89).[74]

This statement reveals the notion of a fear of foreign infiltration. The respective respondent attached a lot of importance to the cultural and linguistic adaptation of the migrant doctors in his hospital. Hence, he expressed a certain discomfort with the circumstances under study.

Although some HR managers and medical directors felt that at the moment of the interview there were again more German doctors on the market (e.g. IP26: 62, IP31: 113), they did not expect that trend to last. On the contrary, they expected to also have to rely on migrant physicians in the future: "[W]e have to live with the fact that we have more foreign than German applications"

---

71 „Die sind froh, dass sie hier sind und geben da richtig Gas. Und die diskutieren nicht lange" (IP31: 111).
72 „[D]as hilft also im Ablauf, andererseits hemmt es manchmal den Ablauf, weil man selber etwas tut, aus seiner deutschen Denkweise heraus, was einem ausländischen oder zugewanderten Arzt völlig fremd ist und erhöht dadurch den Aufwand, das zu erklären oder schürt das Missverständnis, weil das eben schräg ankommt" (ibid.).
73 „[W]eil es letztlich Vorurteile abbaut, [man] selbst den eigenen Horizont erweitert" (IP27: 99).
74 „Also ich kann das nur begrüßen, ne. Wenn die Kulturen zusammenwachsen, dann gibt es auch ein Verständnis für die Kulturen, äh, es muss halt nur jede Kultur die andere Kultur zulassen. Das darf ja kein einseitiges Geschäft werden und überrennen. Also das finde ich schon sehr, sehr wichtig, ne" (IP26: 89).

(IP13: 1179).[75] Therefore, representatives of rural hospitals already decided to further extent the pool of CEE countries from which they seek to recruit migrant physicians by adding Spain in the future (IP26: 64).

While the respondents representing the rural hospitals claimed to be largely satisfied with the incorporation measures they provided for migrant physicians (e.g. IP11: 71; IP13: 187), some of them planned to develop ideas on how to additionally support them in becoming acquainted with their new environment beyond professional matters (IP27: 105; IP31: 196ff.), with the aim to ensure their well-being on-site:

It's important to us that they feel comfortable with us. You've to look at it that way, too. You can't see the physicians as modern slaves, but we ask them to join us, we're in need for them, you clearly have to say that. And therefore, we've to emphasize that they feel comfortable here with us (IP27: 54).[76]

Interviewees representing the city hospitals implied that they would think about the introduction of language classes for migrant physicians (IP15: 72). They were pessimistic about future developments, and expected the shortage of physicians to affect their hospitals to a larger extent than they had experienced so far: "Then it's maybe necessary that we've to change our attitude. Well, we don't have a rejecting attitude, but also none which specifically addresses those applicants" (IP22: 129).[77]

In sum, the respondents were rather ambivalent towards the migrant physicians in their hospitals. While some respondents had accepted the situation and appreciated the enrichment in terms of commitment to work and intercultural competence with regard to patient care, others felt threatened by the cultural difference or identified it as hampering the work routine. In any case, both HR managers and medical directors of the city and the rural hospitals did not predict a foreseeable end to the shortage of physicians, but prepared for a deterioration of the circumstances.

75 „(...) [W]ir müssen immer damit leben, dass wir mehr ausländische Bewerbungen haben als deutsche" (IP13: 1179).

76 „[W]ir legen ja auch Wert drauf, dass sie sich bei uns wohlfühlen. Muss man ja auch so sehen. Man kann ja die Ärzte nicht als moderne Sklaven an-, ansehen, sondern wir bitten die ja zu uns zu kommen, sind ja auch darauf angewiesen, muss man ja ganz klar sagen. Und insofern müssen wir natürlich auch Wert darauf legen, dass sie sich hier bei uns auch wohlfühlen" (IP27: 54)

77 „[D]ann müssen wir uns womöglich noch eine andere Haltung zu dem Thema zulegen. Also wir haben ja keine, keine ablehnende Haltung, aber jetzt eben keine, die jetzt besonders gezielt diese Bewerberkreise anspricht" (IP22: 129).

5.6 Interim Conclusions

The purpose of the present chapter was the depiction of the perspective of the HR managers and medical directors of German hospitals on the recruitment and incorporation of CEE migrant physicians in their facilities. The findings are based on nine expert interviews which were conducted in hospitals in the North, East, and West of Germany in both urban and rural areas. The analysis focused on the process of the recruitment as well as on the perception thereof by the interviewees. The chapter was structured chronologically discussing the reasons for the recruitment of medical doctors from abroad, recruitment strategies and criteria applied by the human resource departments, measures taken to support the migrant physicians' incorporation, and future prospects held by the respondents.

Throughout the chapter a number of tensions and contradictions could be identified. First of all, as reason for the employment of CEE migrant physicians in their hospitals, all HR managers and medical directors named the fact that they were struggling to fill their vacancies with German (-trained) doctors, albeit to different extent. They attributed the main responsibility for the pressing situation to the government and its inactivity in addressing the issue. Their incomprehension and indignation about the lack of measures allowing for an increase of university places, they felt alone with the problem. Interestingly, the alleviation of barriers for migrant physicians to obtain the medical license and thus allowance to practice medicine in Germany, was not acknowledged as a legitimate measure to meet the demand. Here tensions can be identified between the general rejection of the recruitment of medical doctors from abroad on the one, and the dependence on this measure on the other hand. Correspondingly, the recruitment of CEE migrant physicians was not only demand-driven, but on the part of some of the interviewees also perceived as an undesired compromise solution.

As mentioned above, the different hospitals in the sample were affected by the shortage of physicians to varying degrees. In general, city hospitals suffered less from the pressing situation than rural hospitals. Yet, also city hospitals occasionally experienced difficulties in filling vacancies. The degree to which hospitals experienced a shortage of physicians determined all measures taken in order to address the problem, including recruitment strategies, employment criteria, and incorporation measures applied. Whereas city hospitals could still rely on conventional measures to fill open positions with German (-trained) and German-proficient migrant physicians, this was no longer possible for rurally located facilities. They were constrained to become active, and engage in targeted recruitment from abroad by relying on encompassing infrastructures specialised in the recruitment of medical doctors from CEE countries. However, in spite of their suspicion towards recruitment agencies, also representatives of city hospitals admitted to occasionally rely on their services in very pressing situations. This procedure again mirrors the reluctance of the respondents to engage in recruitment from abroad and reveals a rather negligent and short-sighted way of dealing with the problem. These interviewees engaged in ad-hoc recruitment instead of taking care of a more sustainable human resource development.

Feeling compelled to rely on migrant physicians, the HR managers and medical directors intended to find candidates that were as similar as possible to German (-trained) physicians. This applied to professional and linguistic skills, as well as cultural background. While one reason for this preference was the increased efforts in terms of bureaucracy and incorporation that accompany the employment of a migrant physician, further motives could be identified in the protection of local professional standards and cultural values. Both intentions seemed to be transmitted by focusing primarily on German language proficiency as crucial requirement in the medical profession. This requirement served as sign for professional as well as cultural proximity. The fixation on 'the language issue' vis-á-vis individual statements that the German competence is not the most crucial condition (because it was assumed to come naturally over time), implies that migrants' level of German proficiency is used to broadly define other concerns. These range from undesired otherness to a fear of foreign infiltration. This is not to deny the significance of language for an interactive profession such as medicine and the understandable necessity thereof for a smooth daily routine, particularly in times of staff shortages, but to point to a potential overstatement of 'the language issue' in order to express the complications accompanying the recruitment from abroad.

However, striking with regard to perceived likeness was particularly the emphasis of the presumed cultural proximity of CEE migrant physicians to German (-trained) colleagues and the repeated demarcation of migrant doctors of African and Arab, and specifically Muslim background. Unwilling to accept recruitment from abroad in general, in case of doubt, HR managers and medical directors preferred those that they expected to be most alike. This confirms the thesis Favell (2008b) put forward when assuming that the old member states would grant immigration to citizens from CEE countries perceiving them as "lesser evil" than those with Muslim background. These underlying mindsets that are not reflected on impact the HR managers' and medical directors' attitude towards the recruitment of physicians from abroad.

In spite of the high demands expressed on the part of all interviewees, the provision of support on the part of the hospital administrations greatly differed. While almost all of them helped with bureaucratic and organisational tasks upon arrival to enable the migrant physician to quickly take up employment, linguistic, and professional support were offered only to a limited degree. Particularly the acquisition of the highly requested language skills was widely regarded as the physicians' own responsibility. If language classes were offered, these took place off the official working hours in order not to interfere with the doctors' professional responsibilities. This contradiction between stressing the relevance of German proficiency on the one hand, and supporting its acquisition only to a limited degree on the other, speaks well to the implication that initial language skills are overrated and can better be obtained through practical experience. However, it additionally underlines the hospital administrations' perspective of them standing on the supply side, while the migrant physicians are on the demand side. Therefore, the burden of integration was mainly attributed to the migrants. The understanding of the situation as being of mutual interest was rare. Instead, the majority of the respondents had high expectations towards the migrant doctors not seeing the hospitals' advantage of a sustainable incorporation with the effect of having well-trained and well incorporated physicians.

Despite the dissatisfaction with the overall situation, the respondents identified various advantages of the presence of the migrant physicians in their hospitals ranging from linguistic help with migrant patients, cultural enrichment and the chance to broaden one's own horizon, as well as the diligence and zeal of the CEE migrant physicians. The latter matches the statements MacKenzie and Forde (2009) quoted from their interviews with employers in the UK justifying their preferred recruitment of migrant workers. Similar to the HR managers and medical directors, they appreciated the migrants' reluctance to complain as well as their work ethics. This again reveals tensions between a rather restrictive attitude towards the recruitment of migrant physicians on the one hand, and the readiness to benefit from the qualities and skills they bring along.

In a few cases, also the well-being of the migrant physicians on-site was discussed including aspects going beyond work, such as efforts to counteract the risk of social isolation. However, vis-á-vis the consensus among the HR managers and medical directors that in the future the reliance on migrant physicians will remain inevitable, the entire recruitment process including recruitment strategies and incorporation measures reveals a lack of sustainable HR management. The mostly ad-hoc endeavour to fill open medical positions combined with the eagerness to maintain familiar patterns, and the refusal of more long-term oriented incorporation measures do not do justice to the situation.

In sum, apart from few exceptions, the interviewees perceive the recruitment of migrant physicians as a compromise solution, and endorse it mainly from a functionalist perspective putting the hospital's interest first instead of establishing a welcoming culture in their facilities. This attitude neither reflects the rhetoric of a demand of highly-skilled that accompanies the recent liberalisations of immigration policies in Germany, and the facilitated access to the medical license for migrant physicians, nor does it appear as a sustainable strategy vis-á-vis the current shortage of physicians and the respondents' estimation that this pressing state will persist. From an institutional perspective, barriers for CEE migrant physicians to formal recognition and adequate employment have disappeared. However, this chapter has elaborated why they have not entirely dissolved, but rather still prevail in a more subtle way in the attitudes of some of the interviewed HR managers and medical directors.

6 Transferring professional knowledge and skills – the CEE migrant physicians' experiences in German hospitals

After the depiction of the perspective of HR managers and medical directors on the recruitment of CEE migrant physicians to their hospitals, this present chapter portrays the view of the migrant doctors. It presents their perception of the situation and the experiences they have. In order to facilitate the comprehensiveness, the chapter is again structured chronologically matching the different steps of the CEE physicians' migration process. The chapter starts with the depiction of the recruitment and the migration process (6.1) including the reasons and expectations for which the physicians chose to leave for Germany (6.1.1), factors that motivated them to choose Germany as a destination country (6.1.2), reasons for choosing a particular hospital in Germany to work in (6.1.3), as well as the employed migration strategies of the physicians (6.1.4). The second sub-chapter deals with barriers and struggles, the migrant doctors encountered mainly during their initial phase on-site (6.2). These cover the process of acquiring the formal recognition of the physicians' qualifications (6.2.1), language difficulties (6.2.2), differences in the professional order and working culture (6.2.3), problems in the transfer of the doctors' professional self-concept (6.2.4), the doctor-nurse relationship (6.2.5), as well as prejudices and discrimination based on the migrant physicians' national origin (6.2.6). The subject of the third sub-chapter (6.3) is the migrant physicians' reflections on their migration decision as well as their initial expectations (6.3.1), and their weighing of the migration costs with respect to making future plans (6.3.2). Finally, the chapter ends by drawing some interim conclusions (6.4).

6.1 Migration motives and strategies

6.1.1 Seeking professional 'normality' – motivations and expectations of migration

Regarding the reasons the CEE migrant physicians under study reported for their emigration, the findings match those of previous studies on medical migration. Traditionally, low salaries and poor working conditions are seen as the main driving forces for the migration of health professionals with push factors often being more crucial than pull factors for the migration decision (Blitz, 2005; Tjadens et al., 2012). With regard to intra-EU medical migration, this applies especially to migrants from low-income countries such as Bulgaria

(Moutafova, 2011), and Romania (Rohova, 2011). Apart from low monetary rewards, low social recognition for the physicians' work influences decision to leave, e.g. of Lithuanian (Padaigia, Pukas, & Starkienie, 2014) and Romanian (Toader, 2012) physicians.

As shown in the Polish case (Kołodziejska, Makulec, & Schulecka, 2012), economic reasons also apply regarding the working conditions. Accordingly, the underfunding of the health care system in Poland plays a major role in motivating physicians' emigration. Furthermore, nepotism and corruption, as well as discrimination, contribute to the migration decision of health workers from EU and non-EU countries (Tjadens et al., 2012), and a lack of opportunities for specialist training in the countries of origin, as mentioned by medical migrants from various CEE EU and non-EU countries in Germany (Ognyanova et al., 2014). Matching these results, the physicians under scrutiny can also generally be characterised as, what Glinos and Buchan (2014) call, "career-oriented migrants."

At the same time, the findings correspond to insights in the literature on post-accession East-West migration to the UK (see ch. 3.1) in terms of migrants not merely looking for a higher income, but for an income and working conditions enabling them to lead a 'normal' life (Galasińska & Kozłowska, 2009). In the context of this present study, the notion of normality applies to being able to live off one's salary, but especially to professional standards the migrant doctors' perceived as missing in their former work places. Part of these standards was having access to specialist training in the first place, and being free to choose the field and location of residency. In this respect, parallels can be found in the study on the migration of doctoral students from Poland and Bulgaria to Germany and the UK by Guth and Gill (2008). They found that the students did not migrate for a higher income as such, but in order to have the financial means to be able to write a dissertation, and thus to advance in their career by some means. In the same vein, the migrant physicians migrated for the opportunity to complete specialist training.

This motivation applied to most of the interviewees. Eight of the physicians in the sample had started specialist training already before coming to Germany. Out of those eight, one had finished residency in his home country and came as a medical specialist to Germany, another one took the final exam in his home country after having taken up employment in a German hospital already, four of them continued residency in the same specialist field in Germany, and two of them opted for another medical field. What all of them had in common, including those who had started or completed residency outside of Germany, was dissatisfaction with the conditions for residency, as well as for working as physicians in their former countries of residence. They perceived a mismatch between their ideas of an adequate institutional set-up of the medical profession, as well as a medical doctor's role and recognition and the actual realisation thereof in the countries they worked or studied in. The reasons migrant physicians gave for their stated dissatisfaction with the organisation of residency and the working conditions covered several aspects, but did not differ significantly between the different countries represented in the sample.

Restricted access to specialist training

One prominent aspect that the migrant physicians mentioned as motivating their decision to migrate was the way in which places for specialist training were awarded in their home countries. Due to central planning, numbers of places for residency were limited, and the medical field, as well as the location of where to complete residency were more or less determined by the health ministry. Hence, physicians felt restricted in their autonomy to plan their professional career. In many countries, such as in Romania and Poland, in order to complete their studies all medical students had to pass a nation-wide test assessing their performance. Based on the results the candidates were then to choose place and field of residency. However, the available places were limited, determined by a central administrative body, and awarded according to the students' performance in the placement test (Kołodziejska et al., 2012; Rohova, 2011). Those medical students with the best results made their choice first. Consequently, not everyone got the opportunity for specialist training, and those who did could not freely choose the field of specialisation or place of residency. As Dr Gregory House elucidated: "[T]he problem is that you may only obtain a degree or residency at particular central universities – that is, in big cities. The opportunity to receive specialist training in such a hospital doesn't exist. In such a small region and so on (IP07: 4).[78][79]

Instead, graduates were more or less assigned to positions, if the most popular ones were already taken before one got the chance to make one's choice (IP09: 10; IP10: 16). Those who did not manage to acquire one of the rare places for residency could still practice medicine as a general practitioner, or also in their field of interest, but could not advance to become a medical specialist. Therefore, crucial decisions about their own professional future were taken out of the physicians' hands, which motivated them to emigrate.

Low salaries

Additionally, financial aspects in terms of little or no income during residency contributed to the CEE physicians' dissatisfaction. In some of the countries in

---

78   „[D]as Problem ist aber, man darf die Ausbildung oder die Weiterbildung nur in bestimmten universitären Zentren machen. Das bedeutet, nur in der Großstadt. Die Möglichkeit, die Weiterbildung in so einem Krankenhaus zu machen existiert nicht. In einem so kleinen Landkreis usw." (IP07: 4).

79   Since the interviewees are not native speakers, their interview accounts sometimes were grammatically incorrect. In the translations I therefore focused on the content rather than the exact wording.

which the migrant physicians completed their studies, junior physicians in training received no income. This applied to Dr Christa Brinkmann who would have had to cover the costs for specialist training herself, and additionally would have had to move to a city in which living costs were very high. Since she had a family to support, this was unaffordable for her. Thus, she would not have been able to specialise at all and would have had to keep practicing as a general practitioner (IP01: 2).

In other countries, junior physicians received a small stipend instead of a salary (IP05: 6), or had only a small income that would not suffice to live off (IP03: 4). Therefore, Hungarian, but also Polish respondents stated that it would be necessary to have more than one job to earn a living, and to do a lot of additional night and emergency shifts. Accordingly, Dr Martin Stein explained:

Of course, you can do so, but it's very stressful – not because of the job itself, but because of the uncertainty. It may change every month. You either receive no shifts any more or you receive any shift or simply the most unsuitable one, so...yes, it's difficult (IP08: 108).[80]

While such precarious working conditions were regarded as unreasonable by young, single physicians, they were perceived as unacceptable by physicians who had, or were planning to found a family even more so. This was the case for Dr Michaela Quinn. With both her and her husband still being in professional training, both salaries did not suffice to make ends meet for them and their daughter, and to build some reserves. "Financially it didn't work out so well and we were always in the red" (IP23: 10; see also IP02: 2; IP29: 10).[81]

However, Dr Christina Yang, who did not have children, pointed out that she regarded the small income in her home country as inadequate and insufficient for medical doctors. She revealed a certain class consciousness and expressed the claim for a reward adequately representing the high status that she implicitly attributed to physicians, and that she expected others to award the medical profession, too. "It's actually a problem on the government's side. They simply don't understand that we can't make a living with such a low salary. (…) That's impossible. We're doctors, we're not…, anyway, we need some things" (IP18: 225/227).[82] Dr Christina Yang, hence, felt that in her home country she did not receive the salary reflecting the high social status of physicians that she expected as a norm.

---

80   „[N]atürlich kann man es machen, aber das ist sehr viel Stress. Nicht wegen Tätigkeit, aber wegen Unsicherheit. Es kann sich jeden Monat ändern. Man kriegt keinen Dienst mehr oder kriegt man irgendwelche oder kriegt man nur die ungünstige, so... Ja, das ist schwierig" (IP08: 108).

81   „[F]inanziell hat es nicht (gereicht) und äh, das hat dann nicht geklappt, weil das, wir, finanziell war immer, immer dann im Minus, ne'?" (IP23: 10).

82   „[D]as ist eigentlich ein Regierungsproblem und ähm die verstehen einfach nicht, dass, wir können einfach nicht mit einem ganz, ganz kleinen Gehalt, das geht nicht. (…) Wir sind Ärzte, wir sind nicht, naja egal, wir brauchen einige Sachen" (IP18: 225/227).

Lack of resources and medical equipment

Financial resources also played a role with regard to the actual training and working conditions in local hospitals in terms of resources and equipment. Dr Kathrin Globisch, for example, was planning to write a dissertation later on. However, she argued that in her home country there was no funding to develop research. She would not be able to realise this professional aim of hers (IP05: 6). Poorly equipped hospitals were mentioned as another consequence of a lack of financial resources in the health care system. Dr Elias Bähr complained about the lack of modern technical equipment in hospitals in his home country.

Well, you can also notice a process in [my home country], but it is a very slow one. Thus, I said to myself, okay, two years have already passed, and now, I would really like to gain more knowledge, and learn more with new, modern equipment (IP28: 16; see also e.g. IP19: 12).83

Therefore, both Dr Kathrin Globisch and Dr Elias Bähr regarded the lack of resources and modern technical equipment as a shortcoming hampering their own career advancement and thus falling short of their demands.

In a related point, Dr Elena Eichhorn even questioned the purpose of her work if not being able to apply modern standards. She had completed large shares of the clinical part of her medical studies in a German hospital, but worked in her home country for two years before migrating in 2001. When asked about her expectations towards migrating to Germany she stated:

Well, that I can simply realise medical treatment as I've studied it at university. I wanted to put the standards I've learnt into practice. Instead, I used not more than one percent of what I've learnt and received excuses like, "That's not possible, you can't do this, there is no way, it's not approved." I wondered, why then should I work at all? (IP09: 12)84

While in the case of Dr Elena Eichhorn it is ambiguous why exactly she suffered from not being able to put her knowledge and skills into practice, Dr Susan Lewis clearly deplored these same circumstances with respect to resulting deficiencies in medical care. "It was not possible to treat the patients in the best way, and there was no money to provide the best medication" (IP04: 9).85 Hence, she felt like lagging behind advanced medical possibilities in terms of

---

83 „Also kommt schon was in [meinem Heimatland] auch, aber sehr langsam und habe gesagt, 'OK, zwei Jahre ist vorbei ich möchte ein bisschen noch dazu lernen und äh, etwas besser kennenlernen, also mit neue Gerät, moderne Geräte" (IP28: 16).

84 „Na, dass ich einfach die Medizin, die ich im Studium gelernt habe, die Standards die ich gelernt habe, dass ich das ausüben kann. Dass ich einfach die Medizin, äh, machen kann, was ich gelernt hatte. Und nicht, dass es praktisch ein Prozent nur von dem was ich gelernt habe und es heißt, "Das geht nicht. Das kann man nicht. Das gibt's nicht. Das darf man nicht." Und äh, ja, wozu soll ich dann überhaupt arbeiten?" (IP09: 12).

85 „[E]s gab keine Möglichkeit, die Patienten die beste, die beste zu behandeln. Und ja, es gab kein Geld und wir konnten die schönsten Medikamente nicht geben" (IP04: 9).

treating her patients, which contradicts the medical ethos of providing patients with the best care possible.

Corruption and nepotism

Another aspect that medical doctors from Hungary and Romania complained about in particular was corruption and nepotism in the health care system of their countries of origin. This applied to the doctor-patient relationship and, as a side effect, also influenced the training relationship between superiors and junior physicians and to job placement after completion of residency.

Describing how, in his eyes, corruption distorts the doctor-patient relationship in his home country, Dr Mark Greene explained:

The patient pays the doctor and the doctor accepts this corruptive act. And that's completely illegal, very bad and a big problem, because, of course, once you accept the money, the patient owns you and may dictate what they want (IP03: 34; see also IP30: 152).[86]

He clearly outlined his contempt for this practice and the violation of rules stressing the contradiction with his moral standards, as well as his conception of the physician-patient-relationship as the doctor having authority. Hence, the reversion of the relationship undermined Dr Mark Greene's understanding of a physician's role, and thus his own professional self-concept. This was further undermined by his experiences as paramedic during studies.

That was really very bad. You feel just like a dog. Everyone says. 'Do this, do that – And nobody is thankful, nobody says anything at all. And yes, that's exactly why we've decided for Germany, because we had been told that things are a bit different here (IP03: 4).[87]

Moreover, Dr Mark Greene identified corruption as damaging the training relationship between experienced physicians and junior physicians. He explained that the bribery additionally promoted competition between the physicians and inhibited the flow of information from experienced senior doctors to less experienced junior doctors.

---

86 „[D]er Patient gibt Geld für Arzt und der steckt es in die Tasche. Und das ist ganz illegal und sehr schlimm und das ist ein großes Problem, weil natürlich wenn man das akzeptiert, man ist gekauft und der Patient kann alles diktieren was sie wollen und was er will" (IP03: 34).

87 „[D]as war wirklich ganz schlimm. So man fühlt sich als wär ein Hund. So jeder sagt, 'Tu das, tu das' und niemand bedankt, ja niemand sagt nichts. Und ja, deswegen haben wir uns für Deutschland entschieden, weil wir haben gehört, dass hier ist es ein bisschen anders" (IP03: 4).

The older doctors do not participate in training [the junior physicians]. There is a surgeon who knows a lot about a certain situation. He is not willing to share his knowledge, because if two or three doctors have the knowledge, he'll get less money (IP03: 34).[88]

The ideal of experienced doctors teaching and sharing their knowledge and skills with inexperienced physicians was nullified. He did not only perceive this as opposing his ideal of a medical training relationship, but also as potentially limiting his desired professional advancement.

Similar fears were expressed by Dr Gregory House. With regard to job placement after having finished specialist training, he stressed the crucial role that contacts played in finding a position in his home country:

Ultimately, who gets the position depends, well, on one's father actually. The head physician might state: I am really happy with your performance at work. You passed the medical exam and actually, you are an excellent candidate, but the position has already been filled' (...) And then you'd have to start looking for another position and no matter where you look, it'll be really difficult *(IP07: 4/6; see also IP17: 30).*[89]

Hence, he is also apprehensive of the disadvantages this procedure could have for his own career advancement. Additionally, he strongly outlined his disdain for this nepotistic course of action and its discordance with his own values. Not being ready to engage in this procedure he expressed his wish for a meritocratic system: "I wanted to have the opportunity to work somewhere where you say, if you're doing well, you stay and you've the chance to later on get a leadership position. If you're doing badly, you go. I think that's correct and normal" (IP07: 10).[90]

In sum, the main factor motivating the CEE migrant physicians to leave their countries was dissatisfaction with the training and working conditions in their home countries, and countries of training for those who studied abroad. This dissatisfaction included the traditional aspects such as low salaries and limited career prospects. Nevertheless, the purpose of earning more money as such was not decisive. In fact, the search for normality triggered emigration. This normality was indeed based on financial stability for the own career advancement, but was additionally oriented towards modern, professional standards and norms. These applied to both one's own professional and career advancement as well as the provision of care for patients. Hence, with regard to

---

88 „[D]ie älteren Ärzte nehmen kein Teil in der Ausbildung. Es gibt einen Chirurg und der Chirurg weiß eine ganz besondere Situation, er will dass niemand die haben, weil wenn das zwei Ärzte oder drei Ärzte wissen werden, dann wird er weniger Geld kriegen" (IP03: 34).

89 „[I]m Endeffekt bekommt die Stelle wer..., naja, abhängig von dem Vater eigentlich. Also der Chefarzt kann sagen, 'Ich bin sehr zufrieden mit Ihnen, Sie haben jetzt die fachärztliche Prüfung geschafft und Sie sind eigentlich gut, aber die Stelle für den Facharzt ist schon besetzt.' (...) Und dann ging's los, du musst dir eine andere Stelle suchen über irgend-, ist egal wo, ist richtig schwierig" (IP07: 4/6).

90 „[I]ch wollte die Möglichkeit haben, irgendwo was zu machen oder zu arbeiten, wo man sagt, bist du gut, bleibst du und du hast die Chance mal eine Führungsstelle zu bekommen. Bist du schlecht, gehst du weg. Ich finde das korrekt und normal" (IP07: 10).

the migrant physicians' expectations, they identified a mismatch between their institutional conception of 'normality' in the medical profession, and the realisation thereof on-site. They hoped to find these desired conditions after migration to Germany. However, this discontent was a necessary, but not a sufficient reason for most of the respondents to migrate to Germany.

6.1.2 Seizing the opportunity – factors motivating immigration to Germany

Regarding the extensive post-accession migration from CEE, and particularly Poland, to the UK, it is obvious that the liberalisation of migration policies through EU accession has tremendously impacted these migration flows, and the decisions of the individuals to leave. Similarly, in the case under study the current demand of German hospitals for physicians from abroad influenced the decision of the CEE physicians to migrate to Germany. These circumstances were perceived as a window of opportunity by the migrant doctors to pursue their career in a way that corresponded to their conception of the medical profession. They often learnt about this opportunity from former colleagues and fellow students who were already working in Germany. The prospect of being able to rely on their know-how or their own previously gained German language skills and work experience in a German hospital further contributed to their migration decision.

The demand of physicians in Germany as a window of opportunity

The current demand for medical doctors in Germany created a favourable momentum for immigration of physicians that intended to complete specialist training abroad, particularly for those from CEE EU member countries. Commonly reported reasons for immigration were bureaucratic facilitations for the immigration of physicians from EU countries on the one hand, and the set-up of the residency system in the German health care system on the other, as elaborated on above (ch. 2.2.1). Additionally, the migrant physicians were aware of the pressing situation in many German hospitals and the readiness on the part of the hospital administrations to employ physicians from abroad. They learnt about this situation mainly from colleagues who had already migrated to Germany and were practicing medicine in German hospitals. Together, the migrant physicians under study perceived these circumstances as a window of opportunity.

Some of the migrant doctors had made the decision to emigrate without having finally decided on the destination. They weighed up different possibilities before opting for Germany, whereas others immediately chose Germany as a destination country. The former way of decision-making was exercised, for example, by Dr Kathrin Globisch who had already considered migration during medical studies. She weighed up potential host countries such as Spain, where she had already gained some experience during a term of studies abroad, England, and also the USA. In the end she concluded that:

> To get accepted as a physician in Germany was really easy. Here there's a shortage of physicians and thus, you can actually do everything. This might not be true for bigger cities, but definitely in smaller cities you can get almost anything [in terms of specialist field]. Whatever you want (IP05: 2/8).[91]

Hence, the fact that she was free to choose the medical field she wanted to specialise in motivated her final decision, while being well aware of the pressing situation many German hospitals were in, particularly rural hospitals, and the advantages this had for her own career choices.

Others again were driven by the general opportunity of, and facilitated access to, residency in Germany. This was the case for Dr Mark Greene. He and his fiancée had had England at the top of their list, too. However, in the end they also opted for Germany. "Our friends told us, that you can't really complete specialist training to become a specialist in England. It gets easier, if you're already a specialist, but not as a beginner" (IP03: 4).[92] In spite of the EU regulations that were in place to facilitate intra-EU migration, access to the medical profession in England was not easy to gain. This was also experienced by Dr Martin Stein who had left his country of origin for the UK in 2004, right after the accession of the first eight CEE member countries to the EU. His initial plan was to complete residency in the UK. He firstly took up a position as a fee-based physician before getting a position for specialist training. However, he did not manage to get a place in his desired medical field.

> Well, after an unsuccessful battle for two years, I just said: 'That's it!' People had no idea where this was going. 'How should this continue?' Everything was completely unclear. And thus, I thought I will move and continue my career where all my colleagues already are (IP08: 10).[93]

However, this was not the only group of CEE doctors that were attracted by the facilitated access to residency in a German hospital, i.e. those who had toyed with the idea of emigration for a long time and then weighed up or even tried different possibilities. This also applied to physicians who had not thought about migration in general before, but who directly made their decision

---

91 „Deutschland war wirklich einfach zu kriegen (…). Mhm, hier gibt's zu wenig Ärzte und du kannst praktisch alles. Vielleicht nicht in Großstädten, aber in kleinen Städten kannst du fast alles kriegen. Was du willst" (IP05: 2/8).

92 „[U]nsere Freunde haben uns erzählt, dass in England man kann die Facharztausbildung nicht richtig machen, nur wenn man schon ist Facharzt, das ist einfacher, aber als Anfänger nicht" (IP03: 4).

93 „So, mh nach erfolglosem Kampf eh nach zwei Jahre, da hab ich einfach gesagt, 'Schluss.' Da war kein Plan von Leuten, die das Schiff steuern. 'Wie soll das weitergehen?' Alles, alles komplett unklar. Und ich dachte, gehe ich dort, wo meine Kollegen schon sind" (IP08: 10).

for Germany as their only option. This was the case for Dr Gregory House. Not seeing a promising professional perspective as a physician for himself in his home country, he had made the decision to drop out of clinical medicine after finishing his studies, in order to work in the pharmaceutical industry instead (IP07:12). The idea to migrate to Germany, hence, did not result directly from his discontent with the professional conditions in his home country, but he was inspired by a friend and fellow student who told him about the current demand for physicians in Germany.

My friend entered the room and said, "Germany needs physicians. All we have to do is learn the language and we'll immediately find a position". And I replied, "That's a little bit of science fiction. Relax! They certainly are not that stupid to just accept anyone" (IP07: 14).[94]

Again, the demand for medical doctors played a major role. They found information about the formal conditions for obtaining the German medical license and immediately decided to take the opportunity. Although Dr Gregory House had already come to terms with his situation and considered ways of making the best of the circumstances by opting for an alternate career, he was nevertheless open for, and enthusiastic about, the opportunity to practice medicine. "It's true what he said, not as easy as he said, but still not impossible. And we'll get the chance to actually have a career. (…) I thought, 'Now I've the chance to practice medicine'" (ibid.).[95]

In a similar way Dr Christina Yang perceived the opportunity to go to Germany as a way out of an unpleasant working situation. After having been denied access to her preferred medical field, she had specialised in another field and worked as a medical specialist in a local hospital for three and a half years. However, she was not happy with her work, and neither was her husband who had not practiced medicine before, but worked as a medical consultant where he had a better income than as physician. He "said, 'Yes, that's it then. Let's just do it. Let's go to Germany. And you will pursue your specialist training and I'll pursue mine and that's it. Then we'll both be satisfied" (IP18: 229).[96] In Germany, Dr Christina Yang opted for her desired medical field and started residency anew, while her husband also took up specialist training. She had never considered other places as destination countries.

I, personally, said from the start that we'll go to Germany. That's it. Well, no, I never thought about going to France. For instance (…), so many colleagues of mine left for

94 „[M]ein Freund ist reingekommen und er hat gesagt, ,Deutschland braucht Ärzte und wir brauchen nur die Sprache zu lernen und wir kriegen eine Stelle sofort.' Und ich habe gesagt, ,Das ist ein bisschen so science fiction, bleib ruhig. Die sind nicht so dumm und die akzeptieren nicht jeden'" (IP07: 14).

95 „Stimmt was er gesagt hat, ist nicht so einfach wie er das gesagt hat, aber ist auch nicht unmöglich. Und wir haben da die Chance, eine richtige Karriere zu machen. (..) [I]ch habe daran gedacht, ,Jetzt habe ich die Möglichkeit, Medizin zu machen'" (ibid.).

96 „Er hat gesagt: ,Ja das war's dann. Machen wir das. Gehen wir nach Deutschland. Und Du machst deine Weiterbildung mal weiter und ich meine und Punkt und wir sind beide zufrieden'" (IP18: 229).

France as specialists.(...) Of, course, you have to continue with the specialist field, but I never considered going to France, no *(IP18: 423)*.[97]

Again, the main reason was the opportunity to choose another medical field. For her, migration to Germany meant the opportunity for professional re-orientation, and thus the chance for a kind of professional self-realisation.

Migrating irrespective of the demand

However, there were four cases in which the demand of physicians in Germany did not play a role, or at least not such a prominent role. This applied to Dr Elena Eichhorn who took up employment in 2001, to Dr Roland Heilmann who migrated in 2004, to Dr Niklas Ahrend, and Dr Matteo Moreau who came to Germany in 2006, and 2007 respectively. Dr Eichhorn's interest in practicing medicine abroad was based on work experience gained during studies in the hospital she later worked in, and a job offer on the part of the head physician on-site (IP09: 6). Dr Ahrend was also directed to a job offer in the team of a head physician he had previously met during a research internship in another German hospital (IP21: 18). Dr Heilmann migrated to Germany due to his dissatisfaction with payment and working conditions in his home country (IP02: 2), and Dr Moreau decided after an internship in a German hospital that he would like to pursue residency in Germany (IP20: 2).

These four doctors all have in common that they migrated to Germany before the accession of their countries to the EU, and before the demand of physicians had assumed the current proportions. Accordingly, Dr Elena Eichhorn especially experienced severe difficulties in obtaining permission to practice medicine in Germany (IP09: 6). Nevertheless, all four of them resembled the other interviewees in their hope that the organisation of medical work and residency in Germany would meet their expectations in terms of the institutional conception of the medical profession on-site allowing them to have the desired conditions for their career.

Social capital motivating migration decision

As mentioned above, in many cases the physicians' attention was called to the opportunity of completing residency in Germany by colleagues and fellow students who had already migrated to Germany. Hence, social networks in the host country were a crucial factor motivating their migration. Relying on oth-

---

97   „Das war für mich, von Anfang an, ich habe gesagt wir fahren nach Deutschland, Punkt. Also nee, ich habe nie gedacht nach Frankreich zu gehen. Zum Beispiel (...), so viele Kolleginnen von mir, die sind nach Frankreich als Fachärzte (...). Natürlich muss man weiter dieses Fach machen @(.)@ Aber ich habe nie gedacht, nee" (IP18: 423).

ers' experiences and know-how made the uncertainty in terms of what to expect and how to deal with unfamiliar situations more assessable. In that way, the social networks reduced migration costs and risks (Massey et al., 1993).

The fact that a large number of medical doctors from the physicians' home countries had recently migrated and were already living and working in Germany played a crucial role in the justification of the respondents of why they chose to migrate to Germany. Their experiences and suggestions encouraged the interviewees to take the same step. Dr Elias Bähr, for instance, explained that 23 out of 28 former fellow students of his had already been practicing medicine in Germany before he migrated himself. "We saw that everyone is satisfied, and that you may do and learn what you want. And I decided that, okay, if that's what things are like there, I'll also give it a try" (IP28: 20/22).[98] His friends' positive accounts about the training opportunities and their good experiences made him confident that there he would get the kind of training he was looking for. In the same way, Dr Miranda Bailey relied on recommendations of physicians working in a German hospital already. In her case it was her aunt who had been practicing medicine in Germany for 30 years, and enticed her to migrate as well. "She told me that there are so many physicians from [our home country] in Germany and that you've better possibilities for residency here" (IP19: 2).[99]

Social contacts outweighing other decision factors

For some of the interviewees, social contacts even proved to be more important for their decision to migrate and the destination, rather than aspects concerning their career, or those that might even have facilitated their work abroad. This was the case for Dr Meredith Grey who was prompted to immigrate to Germany by a friend and fellow student. She had not thought about emigrating before, but liked the idea. "I thought, 'Wow, how cool, new language, new job, new country, new people – I would really like to do this', and then she said, 'Yes, we can do so together'" (IP14: 2).[100]

Social contacts were also crucial for Dr Karin Patzelt's choice of Germany as the destination country. However, she had considered emigration before and was eager to migrate to France due to her proficiency in French. However, for her the prospect of not having to undertake this step alone was more important than training opportunities and even the fact that she did not have prior knowledge of German. "Many, many physicians from [my home country]

98   „[W]ir haben gesehen alle ist zufrieden, also kann man alles hier machen, lernen usw. Und habe gesagt, ,OK, dann probiere ich auch'" (IP28: 20/22).

99   „Sie hat zu mir gesagt, dass naja in Deutschland kommen sehr viele Ärzte aus [unserem Heimatland] und kann man so besser, also ein bisschen besser die Weiterbildung, also die Ausbildung machen" (IP19: 2).

100   „Ich dachte, ,Pah, wie cool, neue Sprache, neue Arbeit, neues Land, neue Leute', ich würde das total gerne machen und dann meinte sie, ,Ja, wir können das zu zweit machen'" (IP14: 2).

came to Germany and my friends said that they also want to migrate to Germany and then, well, and then I didn't leave for France by myself" (IP25: 8).[101]

Thus, social capital influenced and led the interviewees' migration decisions in two key ways: by providing comfort based on the prospect of desired training conditions, and based on the certainty to have company being able to give advice and support.

Country-specific cultural capital motivating migration decision

Apart from other physicians' experiences driving the migrant doctors' migration decision, the physicians' own prior knowledge and experiences also motivated them to migrate to Germany. Some of the respondents had gained language skills or work experience in a German hospital during previous stays in Germany or another German speaking country. This previously accumulated "country-specific cultural capital" (Weiß, 2005) functioned as additional crucial factors for choosing Germany as a host country.

The experience of previous stays in Germany and having accumulated country-specific cultural capital during that time functioned as additional motivating factors for choosing Germany as a destination country. Those physicians who had gained practical experiences during (research) internships and study terms in Germany could draw on the gained familiarity with the health care system, as was the case for Dr Doug Ross who had completed his clinical traineeship in a German hospital. These experiences made the situation more assessable for him and facilitated his decision. "Well, I knew the German health system quite well. (…) And I knew exactly what I wanted and what to expect" (IP17: 36/38).[102]

Moreover, previously gained proficiency in the German language was a motivation to opt for Germany. Some physicians had already learnt German at school in their home countries, while others had acquired the respective language skills during a previous stay in a German speaking country. The latter applied to Dr Leyla Sherbaz who had worked as an au pair in Germany before her studies. She expected her German language skills to facilitate her acclimatisation to the new working environment. "Well, I wanted to go to a country where I at least understand the language and German, yes, I could understand it already" (IP24: 228).[103]

---

101 „Viele, viele Ärzte [aus meinem Heimatland] sind nach Deutschland gekommen und meine Freunde sagt, dass sie wollen auch nach Deutschland auswandern und @dann@, ja und dann wollte ich nicht allein nach Frankreich gehen" (IP25: 8).

102 „Also ich kannte das deutsche Gesundheitssystem ganz gut. (…) Und ich wusste genau was ich will, und genau was ich zu erwarten habe" (IP17: 36/38).

103 „Also ich wollte schon irgendwo gehen, wo man mindestens ja, weil Deutsch konnte ich zum Beispiel mindestens zu verstehen, ja" (IP24: 228).

To conclude, given the difficult professional situation in the physicians' home countries, and the comparably favourable situation in German hospitals, the pressing shortage of physicians in Germany and the readiness of German hospital administrations to recruit physicians from abroad, triggered the CEE doctors' decision to migrate. Due to the often pressing staff situation, as well as the resulting low access barriers, particularly in rural hospitals, as elaborated on above (ch. 5), coming to Germany was seen to be a feasible possibility. Therefore, the CEE physicians perceived these circumstances as a window of opportunity to be able to obtain specialist training and pursue a medical career in the first place, and in accord with their ideas and conceptions of their profession as well as their desired career path. This was further motivated by the fact that many former colleagues and fellow students were already living and working in Germany, thus providing a certain security and ability to assess the risk of what they would undertake. Furthermore, previously gained country-specific knowledge and (language) skills were perceived as lowering the migration costs.

6.1.3   Choosing a hospital – reasons and considerations

The reasons migrant physicians gave for choosing particular hospitals largely matched their initial migration motives. In particular, they were given access to the training opportunities that they had been looking for in terms of a position in the desired field of specialisation and were provided with comprehensive technical equipment (e.g. IP03: 18; IP23: 20). In this respect, the size of the hospital also played a role since the bigger the facility, the larger the spectrum of specialisations and the more likely that physicians could complete the entire residency on-site without having to move to another hospital to learn further aspects of their field (IP24: 39). However, for other migrant doctors the choice of the hospital was impacted by different, or at least additional, non-career-oriented factors.

For instance, Dr Roland Heilmann accepted the necessity to relocate at least temporarily for parts of his specialist training, since he preferred a small hospital due to his concern about finding his way in a bigger one.

I wanted a smaller hospital, because I have to admit that my knowledge of German was rather limited in the beginning. Thus, I wanted to work in a small hospital, because I thought, getting to know your colleagues is faster there, and this may be more pleasant when you start with a few physicians instead of 300 (IP02: 14).[104]

104   „Ich wollte ein kleineres Krankenhaus, weil ich muss ehrlich sagen, meine Sprachkenntnisse waren sehr grenzwertig am Anfang. So ich wollte in ein kleines Krankenhaus, weil ich habe gedacht, da wirst du die Kollegen schnell kennenlernen und dann ist das vielleicht angenehmer für den Anfang als irgendwelcher großer Koloss mit 300 Ärzten" (IP02: 14).

By opting for a smaller hospital he might have made a compromise at the expense of a fast professional advancement. However, in the long run he regarded this decision as an investment in terms of a quicker transfer and utilisation onsite.

Additionally, it was important to Dr Roland Heilmann that the hospital was located close to the border as this enabled him to commute home every weekend as long as his family remained in his home country. This was also a key criterion for Dr Lea Peters who had applied to several hospitals throughout Germany and got accepted in almost all of them, but then chose the one that was closest to her city of studies. She explained, "[S]ince I studied here, I had a lot of friends and here I'm almost at home. Yes, I can work in Germany, but live in [my home country], so it was easier that way, although the hospital isn't as good" (IP10: 10).[105]

Again, compromises were made at the cost of rapid professional advancement, and again social capital played a crucial role for the interviewees' decision-making. In particular, this also applied to those who migrated together with their partners. They were keen on finding positions in the same facility or at least in hospitals that were located close to each other (IP04: 11; IP18: 23). Being less independent, to some extent they subordinated their professional goals to their private interests, reflecting the current stage in their life-course in terms of having a family and thus being responsible not only for their own needs, but also their partners' and children's needs.

Only in one case a physician stated that the hospital he worked in had been the only option for him. "I didn't want to end up living here, but I had no other options" (IP07: 34).[106] Dr Gregory House would have preferred a hospital in or at least close to an urban area. However, due to the fact that he had not reached the B2 level of German proficiency when he applied, he was only given the chance to study German on-site by a single head physician.

In sum, while hospital selection was often driven by career advancement being the main purpose for migration, some interviewees stated that personal matters were an even more crucial aspect in the choice of their new workplace. In some cases this was related to the physicians' own core family and thus reflected the different stages of the migrant doctors in their life course along with different priorities. However, from the literature (Kovacheva & Grewe, 2015b), as well as from the accounts of the HR managers and medical directors depicted above (ch. 5), we know that rural hospitals are more dependent on migrant physicians than city hospitals. Despite occasional pressing staff situations, the latter mainly manage to fill their vacancies with German (-trained) physicians. Therefore it is likely that rural hospitals were more accessible for

---

105 „[W]eil ich hier studiert habe, hatte ich viele Freunde. Und äh, irgendwie bin ich fast wie zu Hause. Ja, also, kann ich in Deutschland arbeiten und in [meinem Heimatland] wohnen, also war es einfacher, obwohl das Krankenhaus nicht so gut wie da ist" (IP10: 10).
106 „Ich wollte nicht unbedingt hier landen. Aber ich hatte keine andere Möglichkeit" (IP07: 34).

the migrant physicians under study. Accordingly, some of the CEE migrant doctors perceive these remote locations as unattractive as well, but agree to work there for lack of alternatives. Consequently, this institutional context was perceived as an opportunity by some of the migrant doctors who might have been excluded from finding a position under different circumstances.

6.1.4   Getting there – migration strategies

As described previously for post-accession migration (Engbersen & Snel, 2013; White & Ryan, 2008), migration strategies have become more independent and individualised in the case of the CEE migrant physicians under study. There are no structured, government run recruitment programmes the physicians participate in. Instead, they migrate by their own means and also rely on family networks only when these relatives are also physicians. This matches the finding by Csedő (2010) who found that for highly skilled CEE migrants who had migrated to London prior to their country's EU accession, and were positioned at the primary labour market, professional networks proved to be more useful compared to family or ethnic networks in finding employment matching their level of skills. Accordingly, the migrant physicians under study relied on professional networks including former fellow students and colleagues in German hospitals they had met during previous stays. Additionally, they increasingly made use of commercial recruitment agencies.

Altogether 11 out of 21 doctors in the sample found their positions without relying on institutionalised ways of recruitment. Six found their positions by responding to job advertisements and sending unsolicited applications, and five were directed to vacancies through their own professional contacts, or those of friends and colleagues. The remaining 10 physicians in the sample came to Germany with the help of an institutionalised recruitment procedure, two of them met representatives of their hospitals at a job fair in their university city, three of them met representatives of recruitment agencies at such a job fair, and the other six approached agencies either on their own initiative or based on a recommendation from their digital or personal social networks.

The strategies of the respondents to migrate and to find a position in a German hospital largely reflected the recruitment strategies mentioned by the HR managers and medical directors in the previous chapter (see ch. 5.1.2). Hence, they either approached human resource agencies that specialised in the recruitment of physicians, or applied by responding to job advertisements, or in an unsolicited way. Dr Elena Eichhorn indirectly described the practice of recruitment based on institutionalised partnerships mentioned by HR managers and medical directors. Based on a partnership of her medical school with the hospital she later worked in, she had the opportunity to complete different internships in the same facility. Nevertheless, this did not lead to direct employment on-site. This was not inhibited by herself, but due to the fact that at that time, in 1999, legal regulations for migrant physicians were still very strict (IP09: 6).

One strategy that had not been mentioned by the HR managers and medical directors is the recruitment of migrant physicians at job fairs. These are organised in university cities in CEE. At such fairs, physicians met both representatives of agencies as well as hospitals that were looking for physicians to recruit, as Dr Kathrin Globisch explained.

That was about a year ago (…). A company, was not just one company, but rather an event with several companies, like recruitment agencies from Germany, Sweden, whatever... They took my contact information and then they called me or wrote to me, I don't remember exactly, and asked which fields I'm interested in. Then I said rather imprecisely "surgery", I didn't name this sub-specialisation, and they responded: "Do you want this? Look at this page." Then I looked at it, and then I got invited to a job interview (…) while I was still studying. And then they said, "Okay, let's wait until [you've finished your studies], and then we'll hire you" (IP05: 4).[107]

However, the accounts of the respondents again stressed two aspects discussed above. These were, firstly, the crucial role of social capital in also finding a position in a German hospital, and additionally, the conception of the demand of physicians in Germany as a window of opportunity due to the massive recruitment infrastructure that emerged in the course of its increase.

Due to the fact that most of the respondents knew colleagues who had previously migrated to practice medicine in a German hospital, they could rely on their experiences in finding a position in Germany (e.g. IP07: 16). Romanian and Hungarian doctors in the sample particularly reported this. Both groups are strongly represented in German hospitals (cp. table 1) implying that they have a large network to rely on. The internet was a useful source for many physicians. Digital networks as well as online forums served as platforms (e.g. IP07: 14/40; IP29: 22). Hence, by sharing experiences and information, those who had already migrated, for example, recommended reliable recruitment agencies to approach (e.g. IP29: 16), and sources where to look for job offers. However, more hands-on information was also passed on. This was the case for Dr Martin Stein whose friends from university were already in Germany. "They knew how these things work and I also received a little bit of feedback,

107 „Das war so, vor einem Jahr, also Mai 2000... ja ehm, ja ehm elf, war eine Firma bei uns - nicht nur eine Firma, sondern so wie eine Veranstaltung von mehreren Firmen, wie Vermittlungsfirmen aus Deutschland, Schweden, was auch immer und die hat meine Kontaktdaten aufgenommen und dann haben Sie mich angerufen oder angeschrieben - das weiß ich jetzt nicht mehr - und ehm gefragt, was, was für Bereiche mich interessieren. Da habe ich gesagt, ‚Chirurgie.' Diese genau Chirurgie habe ich nicht genannt, aber sie haben dann geschrieben, ‚Möchten Sie sowas haben? Schauen Sie sich die Seite an.' Dann habe ich geschaut und dann habe ich das Vorstellungsgespräch im März gehabt, als ich noch im Studium war und dann haben Sie gesagt, ‚Ok, wir warten noch bis August und dann nehmen wir Sie'" (IP05: 4).

and then I applied for the job" (IP08: 12).[108] Respondents also teamed up with other colleagues who were planning to migrate to Germany. As Dr Gregory House explained: "Well, we were a small group of people who exchanged experiences, and we knew exactly that it's better and safer there" (IP07: 42).[109] Hence, they could rely on country-specific cultural capital that was transferred in the form of the know-how of others. Dr Miranda Bailey could even rely on more direct recommendations from her aunt who already worked as a physician in Germany.

My aunt also searched here. She has a friend working here in this hospital. She also worked as a surgeon when she started and yes, she knew, she had a friend here and talked to him and knew they had vacancies in [my desired specialist field], and well, I applied for the vacant position (IP19: 6).[110]

However, she did not only rely on her aunt in her capacity as a relative or compatriot, but in her capacity as a medical doctor and thus a member of a specific professional network.

As a result of the tight staff situation with regard to medical doctors in German hospitals, a market has developed with numerous recruitment agencies offering their services as has been described by the HR managers and medical directors above (ch. 5.2). Although representatives of city hospitals were particularly suspicious of the quality of the services provided by these agencies as well as their integrity, they had to admit to make use of them nonetheless in very pressing situations. Correspondingly, recruitment agencies were widely used by hospital administrations to fill their vacancies. The CEE migrant physicians perceived this situation as favourable since it facilitated their migration to Germany as well as the process to find employment on-site. Professional networks resulting from the large number of compatriot physicians already being in Germany additionally facilitated their job search, either through direct contacts, or through the transfer of country-specific know-how with respect to the application process. Therefore, the migrant physicians found a situation in which the mere process of leaving their home country to find employment in a German hospital was relatively uncomplicated, as well as being supported and encouraged by the hospital administrations.

With regard to the overall migration motives in terms of motivating emigration as well as the choice of Germany as a destination country, it is obvious

108 „[D]ie wussten, wie das alles läuft, so ich habe auch ein bisschen Feedback und eh, ich habe mich dann beworben" (IP08: 12).
109 „Also wir waren eine kleine Gruppe von Menschen, die Erfahrungen getauscht haben und wir wussten genau, da ist besser, da ist sicherer" (IP07: 42).
110 „[Es] hat auch meine Tante hier gesucht. Sie hat auch eine Bekannte hier im Haus, einen Bekannten, naja. Sie hat auch gearbeitet als Chirurg am Anfang und ja, sie kannte hier, sie hatte hier einen Freund und hat mit ihm gesprochen und wusste, dass es hier einen Platz [im Feld meiner Wahl] gibt und naja, habe ich mich hier beworben" (IP19: 6).

that the migration of CEE migrant physicians to Germany, just as other hitherto discussed post-accession East-West migration in Europe, can be categorised as labour migration. However, this medical migration is not used to quickly earn a certain amount of money for investment upon return to the respective home country, nor to gain experience abroad and to improve language skills, as was found for post-accession East-West migration to the UK. Instead, in most of the cases, the focus is on professional advancement in terms of the next career step.

Looking at the employed migration strategies, they prove to be very individual as also found for post-accession migration to the UK. Migrant physicians did not rely on family networks or migration schemes, but on professional networks either consisting of former fellow students and colleagues, or being commercially run. The fact that the former and the latter were numerously in place, resulted from the demand of migrant physicians in German hospitals. Hence, the current shortage of physicians in Germany was reflected in both the physicians' choice of Germany as a destination country as well as in their migration strategies providing them with favourable conditions for migration.

6.2 Barriers and struggles

6.2.1 Gaining formal recognition – institutional mechanisms of closure

Nohl et al. (2010b) already showed that the formal recognition of professional qualifications is a social process underlying decisions on the part of the administrative bodies that are often perceived as random and obscure (Weiß, 2010, p. 134). While those interviewees who came to start specialist training did not perceive the administrative procedure to obtain the permission to practice medicine in Germany as a barrier, physicians who arrived in Germany prior to the accession of their country to the EU encountered difficulties with the responsible medical association. In line with the findings of Nohl et al. (2010) on the labour market conditions of migrants with legally equal access to the labour market in Germany, migrant physicians wanting to get previously completed years of residency recognised also faced complications and delays.

Formal recognition of professional qualifications after EU accession

When asked about the bureaucratic procedure of acquiring the license to practice medicine in Germany, most of the physicians stressed the perceived ease of the process. This was the case for those who had started medical studies briefly before, or after their country of origin had accessed the EU. Obtaining the medical license was an uncomplicated experience, as Dr Doug Ross stated: "Well, the EU was really a life saver for me. I've received all papers easily" (IP17: 64).[111] When he arrived in Germany in 2007, his country of origin had just entered the EU and the freedom of movement for highly-skilled from that country was still an exemption to the transition regulations. Hence, he did not obtain the medical license immediately, but had to apply for a professional permit that had to be renewed every year. However, after one year of his stay, this was already converted into a medical license. "After one year I get mail and it says, 'You can now work here in Germany without any problems.' I didn't request anything. They said, 'without notice'" (IP17: 64).[112]

Hence, the growing demand of physicians tremendously facilitated the process. This was also the perception of other migrant physicians who benefited from this development. The increasing necessity to rely on migrant physicians thus led to an elaborate information policy on the part of the responsible medical associations facilitating the process for migrant physicians, as Dr Mark Greene illustrated:

[N]owadays you can look up everything online. I think that here in Germany the websites are very well organised, so that you can find information easily. And we looked at the website of the [responsible] state medical association and there everything was described. So, no problem (IP03: 22).[113]

Additional proof of this development towards more open practices and attempts to attract migrant physicians was the provision of help by recruitment agencies. This way, the formal recognition of the physicians' qualifications was perceived as merely a formality as Dr Elias Bähr experienced:

Actually, the agency was of great help. 'Cause otherwise I would not have known how things work here in Germany. I mean, what do I have to translate? Where do I have to go? They organised everything. Medical license and so on, everything. So it was really easy" (IP28: 60).[114]

111 „[A]lso für mich war EU echt die Rettung. Habe ich, Papiere alle einfach bekommen" (IP17: 64).
112 „[N]ach einem Jahr kriege ich Post und sagt, 'Ja [IP17], du darfst jetzt problemlos hier arbeiten in Deutschland.' Ich habe nix angefordert. Die haben gesagt, fristlos" (IP17: 64).
113 „[H]eutzutage kann man alles im Internet und so angucken. Ich denke, dass hier in Deutschland, diese Webseiten sind sehr gut organisiert, so dass da kann man die Informationen gut finden. Und wir haben die Webseite der [zuständigen] Landesärztekammer angeguckt und da war alles beschrieben. So, kein Problem" (IP03: 22).
114 „[D]as war eine große Hilfe diese Agentur eigentlich. Weil sonst ich kann, ich weiß nicht wie hier in Deutschland das läuft. Also was muss ich hier übersetzen, wohin muss ich geben. Also sie haben alles organisiert. Approbation usw., alles. Also war wirklich einfach" (IP28: 60).

Hence, in these cases, the automatic recognition of credentials acquired in other EU member countries, as regulated in the EU directive on the harmonisation of professional qualifications, applied without complications.

Formal recognition of professional qualifications prior to EU accession

These facilitations mark a rather drastic change in the bureaucratic procedure as shown by the cases of physicians who arrived in Germany earlier. They encountered major barriers in utilising their cultural capital, as experienced by Dr Niklas Ahrend. He had finished his medical studies in 1999 and received the medical license to work as a physician in his home country after completing the required year of clinical practice. In the beginning of 2001 he then started specialist training in a local hospital. In 2004, during residency, he went on a 10-months research internship to a university clinic in Germany, funded by a German foundation. Although he enjoyed the research experience, he was also determined to proceed with clinical work abroad in order to continue pursuing his specialist training. However, in the German hospital, he was not allowed to work with patients since, as a non-EU citizen, he was neither entitled to the medical license nor a professional permit. He was only allowed to follow other physicians around akin to *work shadowing* as part of his internship, which he found to be unsatisfactory. Dr Ahrend contacted the responsible medical association in order to obtain the permit to conduct clinical work, but failed at that point.

[T]hat was really weird at that time; they did not understand how I intended to obtain this license. They always asked me, 'Are you German?" – 'No, I'm not German.' – 'Are you married to a German?' – 'No, I'm not married. I studied medicine.' (IP21: 41).[115]

The fact that he was a trained physician did not play any role in the question of whether he was entitled to a professional permit or not. Instead, his nationality and marital status were of primary concern. Dr Ahrend perceived this neglect and the non-recognition of his professional qualifications as a devaluation of his professional status and his cultural capital, and as an offense to his professional self-image. Complaining about the way he was treated, he expressed his disappointment by distancing himself from other people waiting with him in line at the immigration office, stressing the fact that he came to conduct research and to work in a German hospital.

(…) [S]tanding there with all the other migrants who had nothing to do with academia, who came from any region, Africa, Asia, and so on, who simply had problems there in

---

115 „[D]as war damals ganz komisch, die haben gar nicht verstanden, wie ich das haben will. Sie haben mich immer gefragt, ‚Sind Sie ein Deutscher?‘ – ‚Nein, ich bin kein Deutscher.‘ – ‚Sind Sie mit einer Deutschen verheiratet?‘ – ‚Nein, ich bin nicht verheiratet. Ich habe Medizin studiert‘“ (IP21: 41).

their countries. They came due to poverty, or, I don't know, well, we were all lumped together back in 2004 (IP21: 212).[116]

Formal recognition of previous years of specialist training

Although this problem had almost vanished for migrant physicians from CEE EU member countries who wanted to specialise in Germany, doctors who wanted to continue residency in the field they had begun abroad also encountered difficulties with respect to the recognition of their qualifications. While one migrant physician mentioned that thus far she had not found the time to address this (IP04: 177), Dr Elias Bähr stated that the hospital administration did not know how to start this recognition process (IP28: 227). Dr Michaela Quinn, however, was eager to pursue this undertaking immediately. She had already completed two years of residency in a country that had accessed the EU in 2004, before coming to Germany. She wanted to get these years recognised so that she could continue with the third year of residency instead of having to start anew. When signing the contract, those responsible in the human resource department of the hospital pledged that she could do so. They additionally ensured her that she would receive the higher salary she was entitled to due to her advanced stage in specialist training. However, she did not receive the information that she would need to apply for recognition at the responsible medical association, and that she would have to obtain the recognition within six months in order to be paid the respective salary retrospectively.

They absolutely didn't say a word about the fact that only after the recognition I was entitled to the higher salary, or that I have only six months, after six months it can still be reimbursed. They didn't say that at all (IP23: 329).[117]

Dr Quinn felt let down due to the lack of information. She also felt exploited as, nevertheless, she was expected to take over more responsibility than she got paid for. "I was classified as a job starter and I was already doing shifts, I worked just normally, independently and so on and then, for me that was very unfair" (IP23: 130).[118] She perceived this negligence as disrespectful and as an injustice towards her and her professional qualifications, which was expressed in the lack of adequate financial reward for her performance. Additionally, the

---

116 „(…) stehen mit all diesen anderen Migranten, die gar nichts mit der Akademik zu tun hatten, die pff, aus irgendwelche Regionen kamen, Afrika, Asien usw., die einfach Probleme da in deren Länder hatten. Also die kamen weil die Armut da hatten, oder ich, ich weiß es gar nicht, also es, wir waren damals 2004 alle in einem Topf" (IP21: 212).

117 „Die haben total kein Wort darüber gesprochen, dass nach der Anerkennung. Oder ich habe nur sechs Monate zum Beispiel und nach sechs Monaten kann es noch zurück bezahlt werden. Das haben die überhaupt nicht gesagt" (IP23: 329).

118 „[I]ch war eingestuft als Berufsanfänger und ich habe schon Dienste gemacht ich habe schon ganz normal selbständig gearbeitet und so und dann, das war für mich ganz, äh, ein bisschen ähm, äh, nicht Recht" (IP23: 130).

responsible medical association had not shown itself to be cooperative. Firstly, Dr Quinn received absolutely no information with respect to her submitted documents. It was only upon request that she was told that her documents got lost. Yet, the documents were found again, but the medical association was hesitant about recognising the submitted certificate of conformity. They claimed that it did not match the requirements.

[T]hey want that everything is according to the content and range of courses for specialist training of this [responsible] medical association. And that can't be, because actually I'm from abroad (…). And it doesn't work like that (IP23: 41-43).[119]

Again, Dr Quinn perceived this evaluation as unjustified and arbitrary. This impression was additionally amplified by a repeated lack of transparency of the procedure as it continued. Again, the medical association did not reply to her inquiries concerning the progress of the recognition process. Moreover, requests on the part of her head physician had no apparent effect. Eventually she found out that during this period the medical association had indeed recognised the certificate of conformity and she could now be classified according to the tariff matching the stage of her training. Nevertheless, due to the lack of information, and the inflexibility on the part of the hospital in paying her according to her qualifications, as well as the lack of transparency and the thus perceived random conduct on the part of the medical association, Dr Quinn did not feel acknowledged in her capacity as physician.

Due to matters of formal recognition, the full utilisation of her qualifications as cultural capital was impaired. Although Dr Quinn's qualifications eventually were assessed, the fact that she acquired these abroad once again constituted an obstacle to their immediate recognition. This illustrates, albeit in an attenuated form, that the closing mechanisms of the medical association towards foreign qualifications were still in place, undermining the successful transfer of knowledge and skills. In any case, both migrant physicians felt excluded and not recognised in their capacity as medical doctors, which posed a threat to their professional identity and self-esteem.

In sum, the examples show that the interviewees perceived the EU citizenship to tremendously facilitate the bureaucratic procedure for gaining the permission to practice medicine in Germany. Additionally, the migrant physicians under study saw the engagement of recruitment agencies as helpful, as well as the increased information provided by medical associations in the course of the shortage of physicians. Hence, a radical change has indeed taken place in terms of policies regulating access to practicing medicine in Germany which was also perceived as such by the migrant physicians under study. Nevertheless,

---

119 „[D]ie möchten alles, dass es nach äh, dem Weiterbildungsordnung von diese [zuständige] Ärztekammer ist. Und das kann nicht sein. Weil eigentlich ich bin von einem anderen Staat (…). Und das funktioniert so nicht" (IP23: 41-43).

institutional barriers remained with regard to the recognition process of previously completed years of residency which was perceived as indiscriminate and unfair. The inactivity on the part of the medical associations in terms of their information policy implies the continuance of mechanisms of closure towards migrant physicians. In the same vein, the hospital administrations lacking support implies that these are predominantly interested in filling their vacancies, but care less about the migrant physicians' benefit.

6.2.2 Hitting a communication barrier– social and formal aspects of communication

Proficiency in the language of the host country is regarded as a prerequisite for finding employment after migration, and is also indispensable for conducting certain tasks on the job (Csedő, 2008, p. 816f.). Particularly in a highly communicative setting such as a hospital in which interaction with the local population is necessary, language skills are essential as also stressed by the HR managers and medical directors (ch. 5.2.3). However, as they admitted, in pressing staff situations they could not always hold up the criterion of fluency in German. Consequently, the migrant physicians sometimes faced language difficulties in spite of having passed the B2 test of German proficiency, which was required to obtain the medical license. They had problems immediately managing various conversational situations that went beyond those standardised ones in the language class. In this respect, the findings show that the language problem is more complex than often depicted since standardised language tests prove to not be an adequate measure. While they only assess linguistic language skills, the findings point to further aspects impacting communication.

Therefore, I draw on the distinction of a linguistic competence on the one hand, and a situational language competence on the other, made by Bourdieu (2009). While the former refers to grammar and the knowledge of words, the latter implies a familiarity with how people communicate in certain situations, and to language-based customs and conventions. It is acquired and incorporated during socialisation in a certain linguistic context and forms a crucial part of an individual's habitus. Situational competence can also be understood as an "encultured" form of tacit knowledge (Collins, 1993, p. 98), stressing the fact that such customs are formed as local cultural modes as well as cultural modes developed in a certain organisation.

Being unfamiliar with these cultural codes and customs of communication, most of the migrant physicians were initially confronted with difficulties in understanding patients and colleagues, as well as in expressing themselves. This even pertained to those who were already competent in German prior to migration, and had practical experience in its use from previous stays in a German speaking country. Hence, in line with the statement of most of the HR managers and medical directors, many migrant physicians identified the German language as a major barrier to the transfer of their qualifications.

Understanding others

During their initial phase of work in the German hospital, all of the respondents encountered a communication barrier in terms of not being able to immediately follow and understand conversations in German. This was the case, although all of them had passed a German test required for obtaining the medical license. Nevertheless, the physicians struggled with the practical application of what they had learnt in several respects. One major difficulty was variations in pronunciation, which particularly challenged those migrant physicians who worked in regions with a strong dialect. Accordingly, Dr Roland Heilmann who had participated in a German language class after migration realised:

Well, in the language class, there you learn the German language, but all these exercises are in principle made so that you (…) only get in touch with standard German. And here I suddenly come to [a region in Eastern Germany], yes, and there I could barely even understand some patients (IP02: 60).[120]

Other patients were hard to understand due to their health status, as Dr Martin Stein observed: "Some people are also very sick and therefore they can't express themselves very well. Yes, the most difficult thing was the language" (IP08: 32).[121]

Difficulties in understanding were further amplified in situations that the migrant doctors were unfamiliar with. Dr Leyla Sherbaz had learnt German during a previous stay in Germany as an au pair, and thus was very confident in understanding German. Nevertheless, she got distracted by factors impairing clear expression on the part of her conversational partners. The intense situation during surgery in which smooth cooperation and communication were required might have caused additional stress that Dr Sherbaz was not initially used to.

---

120 „Naja, in dem Sprachkurs, da lernt man die deutsche Sprache, aber alle die Übungen sind prinzipiell so geführt, dass man da (…) nur mit Hochdeutsch in Kontakt kommt. Und hier komme ich plötzlich nach [Region in Ostdeutschland], ja und da konnte ich wirklich manche Patienten kaum verstehen" (IP02: 60).

121 [M]anche Leute sind auch sehr krank und deswegen können sich nicht ganz gut ausdrücken, ja. Und eh, ja das war, schwierigste Sache war die Sprache (IP08: 32).

You come into the operating room where you have to get oriented and everyone is speaking German with some weird accent, has mouth protection and you're so completely disoriented, you, "Eh, what? Yes? Again, please, (repeat again)' (IP24: 61).[122]

Expressing oneself

Apart from understanding, the migrant doctors' communication skills were impaired by difficulties in speaking and expressing themselves. In this respect, the contrast between theory and practice was again stressed, for instance, by Dr Christa Brinkmann. In spite of knowing how to express herself in German in general, she noticed that her expressions did not always sound the way that she intended, and did not always transmit the information she actually intended to communicate. Dr Brinkmann explained: "[Y]es of course we pass this exam, German exam, but in reality it's different. There are many, many difficult situations, when we can say something, but we can't well, or I can't express myself well" (IP01: 26).[123]

Certain situations required a particular way of communicating, or a certain tone migrant physicians did not master immediately. This was the case, for instance, during explanatory conversations and medical briefings with patients, as Dr Christina Yang noticed. Since medical expressions are used in Latin irrespective of the official language of the country it is employed in, she did not have problems with the technical language of her medical field. The challenge consisted of 'translating' these into a language that patients and their relatives were able to understand. "[T]he medical words were very easy for me. But @the German words@, like for example, I couldn't explain how a gastroscopy works. In medical language – no problem, but @in German it was not that easy@" (IP18: 293).[124] Furthermore, situations that required more colloquial language, for example when they had to report to the local court or police via phone, were perceived as challenging (IP28: 267). While others also identified talking on the phone as particularly difficulty (e.g. IP21: 63; IP25: 124), the requirement of unfamiliar vocabulary and an unknown communication situation might have amplified their discomfort.

One strategy migrant physicians applied to circumvent the discomfort of struggling to make themselves understood in German was to consult other migrant physicians from their home countries to discuss medical issues and to ask

---

122 „[K]ommt man in den OP, wo man sich irgendwo orientieren braucht und alle reden auf Deutsch, mit irgendeinem komischen Akzent, haben Mundschutz und man ist so voll desorientiert, man, ,Ha, was? Ja? Nochmal bitte, (wiederholen nochmal)'" (IP24: 61).

123 „[J]a natürlich wir machen diese Prüfung, deutsche Prüfung, aber in Realität ist anderes. Da kommt viele, viele schwierige Situationen, da wir können etwas sagen, aber wir können nicht uns gut, oder ich kann nicht mich gut äußern" (IP01: 26).

124 „[D]ie medizinischen Wörter für mich die waren ganz einfach. Aber @die deutschen Wörter@ wie zum Beispiel, ich konnte erklären wie eine Magenspiegelung läuft, auf Medizinisch natürlich @auf Deutsch war nicht so einfach@" (IP18: 293).

for advice (e.g. IP04: 46). As Dr Martin Stein tried to explain, it was not only linguistic understanding that he felt was facilitated when being able to speak in his native language. He additionally implied a different level of common sense when communication with other native speakers in terms of a shared understanding of the situation and the respective communication partner due to a common cultural background and a common socialisation.

Yes, I can explain everything very, very, very well in [my native language]. That's one thing. Mh, I don't know how to explain but sometimes you think that it's my compatriot and yes, it's easier, should be easier. Simply like that. Whether that's right or not, I can't tell, but yes, often, often we talk to each other. Particularly during night shifts, simply because there is less chance for misunderstandings (IP08: 78).[125]

This again stresses the social and cultural aspect of communication, which, apart from linguistic competences, influenced mutual understanding and hampered the migrant physicians' smooth integration on ward.

Becoming familiar with local language practices

The migrant physicians perceived the experienced barriers of understanding others and expressing oneself in the intended way during the daily work routine as a major challenge. The problems did not derive from a lack of linguistic competence, but mainly from a lack of situational competence, which can only be acquired through practical experience over time, as the interviewees realised. They agreed that additional language classes that were partly offered by their employers did not help them to improve these skills. One aspect of criticism was the course's lack of practical orientation as perceived, for example, by Dr Martin Stein who summarised the problem as follows: "[W]hat was taught there was not exactly what we needed. We needed simple things, not standard German" (IP08: 52).[126]

Dr Miranda Bailey received such practical terms and idioms needed for communicating with patients from a senior physician who acted as a mentor for her. He identified her difficulties and helped her with very practical and hands-on support. "[H]e told me several times 'You say that like this with the patients, like this in German' (...) He couldn't speak Romanian, but he helped

---

125   „Ja, ich kann alles sehr, sehr, sehr gut erklären [in meiner Muttersprache]. Das ist eine Sache. Mh, ich kann es schlecht erklären, aber man denkt, das ist mein Landsmann und ja, ist einfacher, soll einfacher gehen. Einfach so. Ob das richtig ist oder nicht, kann ich nicht sagen aber ja, häufig, häufig wir sprechen zwischen einander, im Dienst insbesondere, weil es da einfach weniger Chance für Missverständnisse gibt" (IP08: 78).

126   „[W]as dort gelehrt wurde, war nicht so ganz was wir brauchten. Wir brauchten einfache Sachen, nicht Hochdeutsch" (IP08: 52).

me very, very much. 'You say it like this in English' and I understood" (IP19: 97).[127]

However, not all language difficulties could be solved in this way, since many problems could not be explicated, but could only be mastered over time. This was true for acclimating to different accents, or the pace of spoken language on-site. The way Dr Leyla Sherbaz finally became familiar with difficult situations and could understand communication and instructions in the operating room was through experience.

It was most important to simply learn that each surgeon simply has a different accent and so on. Yes, and to understand them. That was most important. This, this fast language in the operating room and particularly also these technical terms, abbreviations and so on, to memorise them. That's more a practical matter which you can barely learn in class (IP24: 85).[128]

Hence, she dismissed the usefulness of a language class for the acquisition of situational knowledge as depicted above, and instead emphasised the necessity of practical learning. This stance was shared by Dr Meredith Grey who attended another German class after having taken up employment in a German hospital. Nevertheless, she felt that she had benefited more from practical experience than from these lessons. "I can't say that I've learnt German from these 10 sessions. I learnt it simply during the everyday routine. I was always there, I had to communicate with the others, I had to understand. (…) And it simply takes time" (IP14: 76).[129]

This applied also to more subtle aspects of understanding than the pace of spoken language, and technical terms used in certain situations that were identified by the respondents. Dr Lea Peters referred to such implicit understanding, for instance, in the form of humour. A person's sense of humour is one example of how significant subtleties in communication make understanding and expression in a foreign language very difficult. "[T]he patients often made jokes and then I often didn't quite understand and then I asked them to repeat and they repeated, but then I again didn't understand" (IP10: 30).[130]

---

127 „[E]r hat mit mir so ein paar Mal gemacht, ‚Das sagt man so mit den Patienten, so im Deutsch.' (…) Er konnte kein Rumänisch sprechen, aber er hat mir sehr, sehr viel geholfen. ‚Das, das sagt man so in Englisch' und ich habe so verstanden" (IP19: 97).

128 „[D]as Wichtigste war, dass diese, diese einfach mal nur mal lernen, dass jeder Operateur einfach mal so, einen anderen Akzent hat usw. Ja, und die zu verstehen. Also das war eher diese Sache, ne so. Diese, diese schnelle Sprache im OP und gerade diese Fachtermini auch. Abkürzungen usw. irgendwo im Kopf kriegen, das ist eher so Praxissachen, die man schwer bei einem Kurs lernt" (IP24: 85).

129 „[I]ch kann nicht sagen ich habe Deutsch von diese 10 Sitzungen gelernt. Das habe ich einfach in Alltag gelernt. War immer da, ich musste mit den anderen kommunizieren, ich musste verstehen. (…) Und man braucht einfach Zeit" (IP14: 76).

130 „[D]ie Patienten [haben] oft Witze gemacht und dann habe ich oft, das oft nicht so richtig verstanden und dann äh, habe ich Sie darum gebeten ob sie, ob sie das wiederholen können, und die haben das wiederholt und dann habe ich noch mal nicht verstanden" (IP10: 30).

Since such subtle modes of communication are deeply ingrained in the local culture, they could not be studied by the migrant doctors during language classes, nor explicated to them by colleagues. Instead, the interviewees had to incorporate them over time by observing, as Dr Leyla Sherbaz realised:

[Y]ou simply have to get used to it little-by-little, to the way people think. Yes, simply put, different mentality, isn't it? It's not so completely different, but it's simply, you have to realise what kind of humour people have, in which way they speak and so on. And then how the patients react here, how they communicate, what they expect and so on, these are little differences, yes (IP24: 192).[131]

Hence, the findings show that proficiency in the local language is perceived as a crucial challenge in the work routine by the migrant physicians, which matches the statements of the HR managers and medical directors above (ch. 5.2.3). However, this challenge cannot be reduced to linguistic language competence in terms of vocabulary and grammar. Instead, the practical application of what has been learnt in formal settings, and thus informal communication skills, were perceived as problematic. This is crucial, particularly for a highly communicative profession such as medicine in which communication is not only required with colleagues from the same field, but also lay people such as patients. Migrant physicians perceived the partially provided language classes as helpful only to a limited degree. Rather, they felt that they had to acquire the necessary familiarity with the German language, and local features thereof, through practical experience and by being exposed to the daily routine and speakers on-site.

6.2.3 Learning by doing – acquiring procedural knowledge

The EU-wide harmonisation of professional qualifications implies a frictionless transfer of medical skills and knowledge from one member country to another. Nevertheless, Ribeiro (2008) and Wolanik and Boström (2012) drew attention to the remaining importance of culturally embedded practices in the national health care systems in terms of codes of conduct and cultural modes of procedures that made it difficult for migrant physicians to find their way in the new working environment. These experiences were shared by the CEE migrant physicians under study who were initially unfamiliar with the work environment and the professional order in a German hospital. This applied to practical knowledge such as the handling of certain technical equipment that differed from the devices the migrant doctors were used to operating, but also

---

131 „[M]an muss sich einfach mal so ein bisschen gewöhnen daran, wie die Leute denken ein bisschen. Ja, blöd gesagt, andere Mentalität, ne? Das ist nicht so ganz anders, aber es sind einfach, man muss merken so, ja, was für Humor haben die Leute, was sie, welche Art und Weise sie reden usw. und dann, wie die Patienten reagieren hier, wie sie kommunizieren, was sie erwarten usw., sind so kleine Unterschiede, ja" (IP24: 192).

to procedures and ways of conduct that differed from the context in which they had been professionally socialised. In contrast to academic knowledge, medical doctors gain such professional knowledge, particularly with regard to interactive processes, exclusively during practical experience (Daheim, 1992, p. 28f.). These institutionalised modes of operation, as well as the situational knowledge of their application, are crucial parts of a physician's competence that are incorporated over time (Dewe, 1996).

Subtle notions such as codes of conducts can be captured with the concept of 'tacit knowledge.' The term of *tacit knowledge* refers to "the fact that we can know more than we can tell" (Polanyi, 1966, p. 4, original emphasis) and describes know-how which is implicit and cannot be codified, and thus objectified. Therefore, tacit knowledge cannot be transferred independent of its holder, for instance, in the form of instructions. The reason for why tacit knowledge cannot be explicated is because individuals are not fully aware of how they actually operate certain actions, such as riding a bike. We know that we can accomplish the action, we undertake the action with the desired result, but cannot explain *how* we do it. Another reason is that those holding the knowledge are not aware of it, as they acquire this knowledge through the experience of activities in their daily routine. Consequently, the transfer of tacit knowledge "requires close interaction and the build-up of shared understanding and trust among" knowing subjects (Lam, 2000, p. 490). It is attained over time through practical experience and learning-by-doing. Tacit knowledge is personal knowledge, "a cognitive resource which a person brings to a situation that enables them to think and perform" (Eraut, 2000, p. 114), and contextual in that it is affected by its context of acquisition. Hence, getting to know a context or a workplace is not only accomplished through formal inquiry, but mainly through a process of socialisation in which actors first observe, and then slowly participate in the daily routine. Accordingly, the migrant doctors that were particularly satisfied with their incorporation were those who were given time to integrate, as well as a reference person that they could rely on for finding their way. Migrant physicians who were not given this support experienced their initial phase in the hospital as being more stressful.

Differences in professional procedures

Migrant physicians who had not yet gained work experience in a German hospital initially encountered various aspects in the daily routine they were not familiar with. This even applied to experienced physicians who had previously worked in hospitals in their home countries or elsewhere, as in the case of Dr Christa Brinkmann who had been employed as a general practitioner for three years before migrating to Germany. She expressed her observation as follows:

"On the one hand we can say, yes, it's also a hospital — again patients, again ward rounds and so on, but it's different" (IP01: 32).[132] One example was the handling of the technical equipment in the German hospitals. Upon arrival migrant physicians were confronted with technical devices they were unfamiliar with and which they had not been using before. This was outlined by Dr Elias Bähr who had worked in his medical field for two years in a hospital in his home country, and who had gained additional work experience abroad during a previous stay in another Western EU country. "Well, this touchscreen ventilator was totally new to me. Of course we also had one in the intensive care unit, also anaes-, and intensive therapy ward, but not in [my field]. That wasn't easy" (IP28: 80).[133] He had similar experiences with the use and prescription of medication, since the names of the medication used on-site differed from the ones he knew from his home country. "The active substance is almost the same, but the drugs have different names, so that you really have to learn, practice how the company [is called] and so on" (IP28: 64).[134]

A more subtle aspect that the respondents noticed to be different in their daily routine was in the performance of medical procedures. For instance, certain medical treatments and interventions slightly varied between German hospitals and those in the physicians' country of origin. For example, this was noticed by Dr Michaela Quinn who had already completed two years of specialist training in her medical field before coming to Germany. "[T]hat was all new for me. Actually, anaesthesia, the initiations that is all the same. But every hospital has its own standards and rules and I first had to get used to that" (IP23: 88).[135]

Bureaucratic procedures were also identified as differing by the migrant doctors, as pointed out by Dr Roland Heilmann, who had worked several years as a junior physician in a hospital in his home country before migrating to Germany.

[T]he documentation is also a little different, yes, the health insurance system is different — this division, accident at work, what is accounted for through the physician, and

132   „[V]on einer Seite, können wir sagen, ja, dort ist auch Krankenhaus, wieder Patienten, wieder Visite und so, aber ist eh verschiedene" (IP01: 32).

133   „Also mit dieser Touchscreen Beatmungsgerät, also wir hatten natürlich auch auf Intensiv normal, also auch Anäs- und Intensivtherapiestation, aber nicht bei uns in [in meinem Feld]. Das war ganz neu, also (3) war nicht einfach" (IP28: 80).

134   „Wirkstoff ist fast gleiche, aber, aber verschiedene Medikamentennamen. Also das muss wirklich lernen, üben wie Firma [heißt] usw." (IP28: 64).

135   „[D]as war alles neu für mich. Eigentlich die Narkose, die Einleitungen das ist alles gleich. Aber jedes Krankenhaus hat ihr Standards und ihre Regeln und daran musste ich mich erst mal so gewöhnen" (IP23: 88).

what through the insurance companies, what is not covered by insurances and so on (IP02: 58).[136]

Additionally, he realised that the bureaucratic effort with respect to explanations that patients were provided with, and seeking their consent, was more extensive than what he was used to (IP02: 69). IP05 shared this impression:

Too many documents, forms and so on, the explanatory meetings for surgeries and so on. We don't have anything like that. The head physician or the senior physician comes and says, 'Tomorrow we'll do the surgery. Okay?' – 'Yes.' So that was that. But here, signature, explanations, signature, another signature, another signature *(IP05: 16)*.[137]

Tacit differences in the professional order

The bureaucratic procedure Dr Kathrin Globisch described with regard to explaining examinations and medical interventions to patients can be explicated and codified once those holding it are aware of it. At the same time she referred to an aspect of tacit knowledge that cannot be explicated, i.e. a different conception of the physician-patient relationship between her home country and Germany. While in the former a paternalistic physician-patient relationship seems to be in place, the latter seems to be oriented towards an independent and informed patient. This is confirmed by Dr Matteo Moreau who made the same observation. "Here they treat the patients more carefully. It's much more considered what they say, and what they want, and their wishes are met" (IP20: 51).[138]

Additionally, the relationship between nurses and doctors were experienced as different by the respondents with regard to the organisation of work and the cooperation between nurses and doctors. For Dr Susan Lewis, this found expression in the ward rounds. "Yes, here [we] work together with the nurses. So we do the ward round together, and in [my home country] I should do the ward round by myself" (IP04: 85).[139] This arrangement additionally reveals a different organisation and nature of the physician-nurse relationship that Dr Lewis was unfamiliar with.

---

136 „[D]ie Dokumentation ist auch ein bisschen anders, ja, das Krankenversicherungssystem ist anders, ja diese Teilung Arbeitsunfälle, was über den Arzt geht und was über Kassen geht, Privatleistungen usw." (IP02: 58).

137 „Zu viele Dokumente, Formulare und so das, die Aufklärungen für Operationen und so. Wir haben sowas gar nicht; der Chefarzt oder der Oberarzt oder der Facharzt kommt und sagt, ‚Morgen die OP. Einverstanden?' – ‚Ja.' Also das war es. Und hier Unterschrift, Aufklärung, Unterschrift, noch eine Unterschrift, noch eine Unterschrift" (IP05: 16).

138 „Hier wird dann auch sehr vorsichtiger mit den Patienten umgegangen. Da wird viel mehr geachtet was die sagen und was sie wollen und den Wünschen nachgegangen" (IP20: 51).

139 „Ja, hier arbeiten [wir] zusammen mit Krankenschwester. Also wir machen zusammen Visite in dieser Station und in [meinem Heimatland] sollte ich allein Visite machen" (IP04: 85).

Another aspect with regard to the cooperation between nurses and doctors that was mentioned by many interviewees was the division of responsibilities between the two professional groups. Again, this is not only about the factual procedures and responsibilities, but also the underlying conception of the doctor-nurse-relationship, as Dr Christina Yang pointed out when elucidating the common division in a hospital in her home country. "[H]ow things work in the hospital is clearly different. For example all i.v., intravenous therapy is not done by the physicians, but the nurses, and it's a bit different, yes, well how things work in a hospital" (IP18: 27).[140] Therefore, differences were identified with respect to the classifications of responsibilities as minor or major tasks depending on who is in charge. As is further elaborated on below, the division of responsibilities was subject to a number of conflicts between migrant physicians and local nurses (see ch. 6.2.5).

Explicating tacit knowledge

In contrast to the "encultured" tacit knowledge (Collins, 1993) of the social component of communication practices, and the relationship between physicians and patients, or physicians and nurses, in the cases of professional procedures and codes of conduct the knowledge can be explicated once those holding it become aware of it. One possibility for gaining an awareness of this kind of knowledge is through the occurrence of some disturbance in the normal procedure (Eraut, 2000, p. 118). In the case under study, this applies, for instance, when someone does not adhere to the implicit rules, such as migrant physicians who are unfamiliar with the habits on-site and thus attract attention when they do not act according to the rules. This irritation then causes the holders of the knowledge to reflect upon it, which enables them to explicate. Another option for attaining this knowledge is by one's own experiences, i.e. through implicit learning (ibid.). Having gone through the same or similar situations, other migrant physicians were aware of the differences and difficulties that physicians who had recently arrived in Germany might encounter. Hence, a factor for the migrant physicians that tremendously facilitated becoming familiar with the local professional order and the local work culture was the help and support of their compatriots and other migrant doctors on-site.

Hence, when Dr Roland Heilmann took up employment in a German hospital in 2004, he was one of the first migrant physicians to arrive in that hospital. His German (-trained) colleagues had not been aware of potential difficulties as all physicians working on-site had thus far been socialised in the same system, and had internalised the same procedures and codes of conduct. Dr Heilmann explained:

---

140 „[W]ie es läuft im Krankenhaus ist deutlich anders. Weil zum Beispiel alle IV, alle intravenöse Therapie das machen nicht die Ärzte, das machen die Schwestern und ist ein bisschen anders, ja, also wie es geht in einem Krankenhaus" (IP18: 27).

I think at that time, the problem was also that my boss didn't know exactly how to deal with that, yes? (…) [T]hey observed, what is he going to do, and how is he going to do it. Also the boss himself certainly didn't know about these differences, yes? (IP02: 108).[141]

These circumstances changed with the increasing number of migrant physicians. Local doctors gained experiences in dealing with doctors who had been socialised in a different health system and were able to identify common challenges. Consequently, they were able to explicate what they were doing and how, in order to pass it on to others. This was experienced by Dr Christina Yang who had already practiced in her medical field in her home country, but then started specialist training anew in a different field when coming to Germany.

[M]y senior physicians told me right from the beginning what I should learn before the first night shift and what I should really know (…). So they already told me: 'You first have to learn that and that and that.' So yes, yes they already had experience with foreigners and they knew the differences between the countries and ehm, they were great, well, they really helped me (IP18: 106).[142]

Due to this extensive initial incorporation, Dr Yang then felt confident in facing the tasks that she had to accomplish in her new position. The support helped her to quickly become familiar with her new work environment and after a short time she was ready to take over full responsibility on ward. "[I]n two months I was completely fit @(.)@. And I could simply do everything" (IP18: 106).[143]

Other respondents benefitted from the fact that there were many other migrant physicians in the hospitals whom they could approach. Sharing the experience of arriving in a work environment where everything is new and unfamiliar, a colleague was able to explicate certain procedures to Dr Susan Lewis, as she stated: "It was very nice @(.)@, because I met this Macedonian colleague and she knew already which difficulties I will have. So, she could tell me a lot, help me a lot" (IP04: 29).[144] This active induction of the migrant physicians facilitated their initial phase on ward for them. Additionally, the hospital administration benefited from this support, since it enabled migrant doctors

---

141 „Ich glaube, damals gab es auch das Problem, auch mein Chef wusste nicht genau, wie er damit umgehen sollte, ja? (…) [D]ie haben so geguckt, was wird er jetzt machen und wie er das machen wird, aber… Auch der Chef selbst wusste sicher nicht über diese Unterschiede, ja?" (IP02: 108).

142 „[M]eine Oberärzte, also wir haben immer gesprochen, was soll man lernen vor dem ersten Dienst und soll man richtig wissen (…). Also ich hatte, die haben mir schon gesagt: ‚Sie müssen das lernen zuerst und das und das und das.' Also ja, ja die hatten schon Erfahrungen mit Ausländern und die wussten die Unterschiede zwischen die Länder und äh die waren super, also, die haben mir richtig geholfen" (IP18: 106).

143 „[I]n zwei Monaten war ich komplett fit @(.)@. Und ich konnte einfach alles machen" (IP18: 88).

144 „Es war sehr schön @(.)@, weil ich diese mazedonische Kollegin getroffen hab und sie wusste schon welche Schwierigkeiten ich haben werde. Also eh, sie konnte mir viel sagen, viel helfen" (IP04: 29).

to take over their responsibilities within a short time, while others had to slowly appropriate local customs by themselves.

Implicit learning

The interviewees were not all provided with knowledge about codes of conduct in such an explicit and targeted way. In these cases, migrant physicians had to acquire the knowledge implicitly, i.e. learning-by-doing. Some migrant physicians felt that they would have greatly benefited from these differences being codified in some form. This was the case for Dr Mark Greene who had realised on-site, that physicians place a catheter in a slightly different way than is done in his home country where he had worked temporarily in a local hospital while studying medicine. "If you collect such practical knowledge a bit better, that would... That, but that doesn't exist and it shall not exist. You've to learn all this yourself" (IP03: 154).[145]

Since such help was not available, the respondents either approached their colleagues with questions informally (e.g. IP20: 14), or in some cases could rely on institutionalised mentoring relationships that had also been mentioned by the HR managers and medical directors above (see ch. 5.4.3). The interviewees differed considerably in their evaluations of the effectiveness of these mentoring arrangements. Dr Leyla Sherbaz, for instance, enjoyed this way of professional incorporation. With time, and without pressure she was given the opportunity to slowly get accommodated and absorb procedures and codes of conduct on-site. "[I]n the beginning you could just walk around with another specialist [in my field] who simply explained the things and yes, then you slowly started to work on your own somehow" (IP24: 81).[146]

However, other migrant physicians did not have such close guidance, but had to acquire the required knowledge with their own initiative. This was the case for Dr Gregory House who was less satisfied with his colleagues' help. After the mentor, he was initially assigned to, had left, he felt that the other colleagues were not as capable in guiding him. Therefore he had to develop his own strategy of how to appropriate the necessary skills and knowledge. He observed his colleagues and learnt from imitating their ways of conduct, which he described as follows: "And I had to, if I may say so, steal everything" (IP07: 119).[147] Naturally, this way of learning took more time than when being instructed by others.

---

145 „Wenn man solche praktischen Kenntnisse ein bisschen besser zusammen sammelt, wäre... Das, aber sowas gibt's nicht und soll's nicht geben. Das soll man selber lernen" (IP03: 154).

146 „[M]an konnte am Anfang mal so einige Zeit nur rumlaufen und mit gucken mit einem anderen [aus meinem Fach], ja. Äh, der einfach mal die Sachen erklärt hatte und ja dann hat man so langsam angefangen alleine irgendwie zu arbeiten" (IP24: 81).

147 „Und ich musste alles, wenn ich so, wenn ich mich so ausdrücken darf, alles klauen" (IP07: 119).

Another strategy that physicians relied on, who received little guidance from colleagues and superiors, was to draw on their own experience of former cases as well as their medical expertise.

You must think, "OK, how do I do this?", "How should that work?" – "Logically it is like that and that and that." And then you do it, yes? The most important thing is to not endanger the patient and yourself, yes? If you pay attention to that nothing bad can happen and you can try different things (IP08: 48).[148]

This rather experimental way of learning also takes longer than direct instructions, and additionally might endanger the patients.

In sum, upon arrival in the German hospitals, the interviewees realised that there are numerous subtle aspects in which the codes of conduct and working procedures on-site differed from those they incorporated in their countries of origin. However, as the HR managers and medical directors stated above (see ch. 5.4.3), most of them did not provide the migrant doctors with any measures to support their professional incorporation. Hence, while some aspects could be actively learnt once they were aware of them, others could only be internalised over time. The process of becoming familiar with the local rules and procedures was facilitated for some migrant physicians with the help of colleagues. While physicians who benefited thereof felt confident practicing independently after a short time, those who had to appropriate these notions by themselves took longer and were more insecure about how to handle certain situations, which, not least of all, could be to the detriment of the patients.

6.2.4 Transferring the professional self-concept – professional role expectations

As argued above, the acquisition of tacit knowledge both with respect to German language proficiency and professional skills and knowledge can only be accomplished through practical experience, and thus must occur over time. Therefore, migrant physicians were not able to immediately assume full responsibility that was bound to their function in the respective hospitals. While still learning, they encountered barriers limiting their scope of action, and oftentimes had to rely on colleagues and other hospital staff to help them out. Hence, they did not manage to entirely fulfil the role of a physician as they had envisioned it. Since the medical profession is characterised by a high commitment of its members to their profession and work (Helmreich & Merritt, 2008, p. 30ff.), and a high degree of professional identity (Dollinger & Hohl, 1989,

---

148 „Man muss denken, ‚Ok, wie mache ich das?‘, ‚Was mache ich noch?‘, ‚Wie soll das laufen?‘ – ‚Logisch ist so und so und so.‘ Und dann macht man, ja? Und eh, das Wichtigste ist, dass man nicht Patient und sich gefährdet, ja? Wenn man das beachtet, kann nichts Schlechtes passieren, kann man dann, verschiedene Sachen dann (ausprobieren)" (IP08: 48).

p. 445f.), the migrant physicians perceived this incapability as a threat. It contradicted their overall positive self-concept, i.e. "(...) self-evaluations that people apply to their capabilities contrasted with reference groups such as professional peers" (Helmreich & Merritt, 2008, p. 30). Both the language barrier and the initial lack of work experience in a German hospital undermined this aspiration, and impeded the transfer of the migrant doctors' professional self-concept. Their disappointment found expression in two different sentiments, which can be described as a "sense of incompetence", and a "lack of autonomy." Threatening their professional identity, both sentiments caused an uncertainty for the migrant physicians, which they compensated for by attempting to adapt to the situation in order to meet own as well as colleagues' expectations and thus, restore their self-concept. This coping strategy can be described with the concept of "protective action" as suggested by Zinn (2004) which serves to prevent uncertainty, or in this case, establish certainty. The CEE migrant physicians did so by assuming the main responsibility for finding their way, rather than relying on others to help them. Once mastering their tasks in an independent way, the migrant physicians gained self-esteem.

Sense of incompetence

Realising that language classes and previous German language skills did not equip them with immediate and frictionless communication in the German hospital, migrant physicians felt uncomfortable and insecure with respect to daily interactions on ward. Not being able to express themselves in an elaborate way and not always understanding their dialogue partner restricted them in their ability to act, and thus to some extent, in their maturity. This left them with a feeling of insufficiency, and a sense of incompetence, as these attributes strongly contradicted their actual expectation of a medical doctor's role. The perceived agony with this condition can be explained with the observation of Helmreich and Merritt (2008) that a professional culture of invulnerability, stressing one's own competence and not allowing for human weakness can become manifest in the physicians' self-concept (ibid., p. 35). Consequently, and matching the findings of Shuval (2000) and Bernstein (2000), the CEE physicians under study experienced their migration as a threat to their professional identity that questioned their competence, which is central to their self-image as a medical doctor. Again, this sentiment has two components: one that refers to the perception of shortcomings towards their self-esteem, and another that refers to the perception of shortcomings vis-á-vis the patients who are not able to trust in the respondents' competences as physicians.

The latter is also a crucial part of a medical doctor's professional identity, since the physician-patient relationship is based on trust. Patients rely on physicians' competences based on trust, as they are not able to assess their actual skills and knowledge in a first encounter (Di Luzio, 2005). Accordingly, they have to rely on the physician to fulfil their expectations towards a medical doctor's role. In her interactionist approach to professions, Pfadenhauer (2003) describes nonconformities between a patient's expectations and the physician's behaviour as the lack of *competence to represent competence* ("Kompetenzdarstellungskompetenz"). Acting competently requires professionals to know the relevant structures and processes, conditions and factors of the work environment, as well as to have the situational and cultural competence to deal with the local circumstances (ibid., p. 118). Professionals receive a patients' trust when they convey the impression that they have mastered the situation and firmly adhere to certain routines and ways of expressing themselves that are expected from them in their respective role. Therefore, on the part of the migrant physicians, a competent appearance was perceived as a crucial measure for their successful incorporation on ward.

Dr Martin Stein who had gained two years of work experience in England before re-migrating to Germany remembered a situation in which he could not understand what a patient was saying since he was speaking with a strong dialect. Therefore, a nurse who was assisting him helped him out repeating what was said in a way that Dr Stein understood. However, although this solved the problem so that he could make progress in treating the patient, he was unhappy with the situation. He was worried about losing countenance in front of a patient who could presumably consider him as incompetent as he had to rely on a nurse to be able to handle the situation. This twisted the usual hierarchy between nurses and physician. As the physician he should have been the one who controlled the situation. He should not have had to ask a staff member in a lower position to help him as this put his authority and capability into question. "It isn't nice if you're asking the nurse in front of a patient what he has actually said, yes?" (IP08: 54).[149]

A similar sentiment was expressed by Dr Mark Greene. He had already started studying German in his home country one and a half years before finally migrating to Germany. Nonetheless, he encountered difficulties in understanding spoken German upon arrival in Germany.

Yes, I was afraid of course, because I can't understand [the regional] dialect very well and there were patients, and also one senior physician – he's a really nice senior physician, but I couldn't understand a word of what he said. And it's really bad when you feel so stupid and dumb *(IP03: 26).*[150]

The expression of his discomfort in the form of fear reveals the severity of his shame vis-à-vis the situation. The embarrassment was based on his feeling of

---

149 „Das ist nicht schön, wenn man vor Patient Schwester fragt, was eigentlich er gesagt hat, ja?" (IP08: 54).

150 „Ja, man hatte Angst natürlich, weil [der regionale] Dialekt, das kann ich nicht so gut verstehen und es waren da Patienten und auch ein Oberarzt, der ist sehr netter Oberarzt, aber ich konnte kein Wort verstehen, was er gesagt hat. Und es ist sehr schlimm, wenn man sich so blöd und dumm fühlt" (IP03: 26).

not meeting expectations posed towards him, i.e. responding, and thus engaging in the conversation or following instructions. Therefore, he was left with the feeling of incompetence.

Dr Leyla Sherbaz, a young physician with a good account of German due to her previous stay in Germany as an au pair, found herself in a similar situation and was also initially intimidated. She felt uncomfortable when having to talk to patients. "[Y]ou're so afraid to talk to the patient, because (3) you simply feel so embarrassed that you don't have such a good language level, yet" (IP24: 73/75).[151] Hence, she put high demands on herself to not only be able to express herself, but additionally to do so in an elaborate way. This demand seems to correspond to her idea of the role and the appearance of a physician. Hence, not being able to understand and to express themselves in the desired way, migrant doctors perceived themselves as lacking crucial features in order to be viewed as professional.

Dr Meredith Grey further specified this feeling of uneasiness.

If you don't know the language and you want to talk to a relative, I personally find that difficult, you don't look competent and that's very important in our job, because people are so sensitive. They reproach a lot and you can also understand why. That's very difficult for me (IP14: 34).[152]

On the one hand, she again stressed the importance of a competent appearance for the role of a physician, and thus emphasised her own demands she was willing to meet. On the other hand, she also referred to the patients' relatives who were reproachful. Thus, she revealed additional expectations she was eager to satisfy. However, by expressing her understanding for the relatives' attitude, she again underpinned her own identification with these role expectations.

The same applied to Dr Lea Peters who had the impression that patients would not trust her due to her lack of proficiency in the German language. "That's not good when the patient comes and can't trust the physician. I understood that, I wouldn't have wanted that either in their place" (IP10: 32).[153] She realised that she still lacked the 'competence to represent competence' (Pfadenhauer, 2003), the ability that is crucial to establish a trustful physician-patient-relationship. Since the respondent understood a competent appearance as a critical aspect defining their role as physicians, this perceived lack of trust was hard to bear for the migrant physicians, as expressed by Dr Gregory

151 „[M]an hat so diese Angst mit dem Patienten zu reden, weil (3) man einfach mal so, (...) Man fühlt sich peinlich, dass man einfach nur so, noch nicht das gute Sprachniveau hat" (IP24: 73/75).

152 „Wenn Du die Sprache nicht kennst und mit ein Angehöriger sprechen möchtest, ich finde persönlich das ist schwierig, man sieht nicht kompetent aus und das ist in unsere Beruf ganz wichtig, weil die Leute sind so empfindlich, die machen so viele Vorwürfe und kann man auch verstehen warum. Das war für mich schwierig" (IP14: 34).

153 „Das ist nicht gut wenn der Patient kommt und er kann dem Arzt nicht vertrauen und dann, ich habe das aber verstanden, ich wollte das ähm, äh, an ihrer Stelle auch so, nicht so richtig" (IP10: 32).

House. "That was horrible in the beginning. (…) [W]hen you see in their eyes that they're feeling so bad and insecure, and are always asking themselves, 'Does he understand me? Doesn't he understand me?'" (IP07: 166). [154]

Hence, migrant physicians perceived themselves as incompetent, not being able to meet their own expectations towards their role as medical doctor, and suffered from not being able to create trust on the part of the patients. They initially failed in transferring their professional self-concept to their new working environment, which was perceived by them as threatening their professional identity.

Lack of autonomy

The communication barrier, as well as a lack of work experience in a German hospital did not only hamper the migrant doctors' transfer of their professional self-concept in terms of a sense of incompetence. They additionally required them to frequently rely on colleagues and other hospital staff, such as nurses, to help them out when they did not know how to proceed. This dependency caused them additional discomfort as it undermined their individual clinical autonomy, i.e. "the responsibility for decisions taken in treating the patient" (Allsop & Mulcahy, 1998, p. 77; see also Freidson, 1970). Since clinical autonomy is an entrenched norm and thus a crucial part of the medical professional order, the initial lack thereof impeded the migrant physicians' self-esteem as medical doctors. Again, this notion had two components: expectations the migrant physicians had towards themselves, and expectations they perceived their colleagues to have towards them.

Meeting one's own expectations

Dr Theresa Koshka had completed residency in her country of origin, and had worked there as a medical specialist for two years before coming to Germany. She had gained significant medical competence and expertise, but was hampered in applying it in the German hospital she worked due to language difficulties. Therefore, she perceived her actual capability to be restricted since she had the medical knowledge and know-how, but missed the linguistic and situational competence to apply her skills. This impaired her capacity to act, and slowed down the work process. "[I] know that I can do my work very, very well. There is just this, what is it called? (…) Barrier? When something stops" (IP30: 102/104).[155]

---

154 „[W]ar schrecklich am Anfang. (…) [W]enn man in den Augen sieht, dass, dass die sich so schlecht und unsicher, sich so fühlen und sich die Frage immer stellen ‚Versteht der mich? Versteht der mich nicht?'" (IP07: 166).

155 „[I]ch weiß, dass ich kann meine Arbeit sehr, sehr gut machen. Es gibt nur diese (3) weiß nicht wie heißt... (…) Hürde? Wenn etwas stoppt" (IP30: 102/104).

Some migrant physicians regarded their inability to fulfil their tasks to the extent and at the pace they were used to as their own shortcoming, and that they were responsible to rectify these shortcomings by themselves. Accordingly, Dr Susan Lewis did not note her overtime, nor in any other way request to be disburdened, but regarded the extra hours she took in order to manage the work load as the result of her own insufficiency. "Well, it's my problem that I shall do extra hours, because I've less experience" (IP04: 133).[156]

Dr Matteo Moreau who felt particularly overwhelmed with bureaucratic tasks such as writing discharge letters and doing other paper work, also worked extra hours as he did not manage to complete these tasks within working time. As with Dr Susan Lewis, he was inclined to manage the work load alone, even if that meant doing work after the official hours.

Now, I usually write a discharge letter in three to five minutes, but at that time it took me 30 minutes. And that doesn't work when it takes me six, five, six hours @sitting here, or more@ for 10 people. I then did that at home (IP20: 32).[157]

This endeavour was motivated by the ideal of self-sufficiency and autonomy as characteristic for the physician's role that the respondents were keen to match. For instance, Dr Martin Stein's initial dependence was not compatible with his self-image of an advanced junior physician who had previously gained approximately two years of work experience in England. Accordingly, Dr Stein justified his refusal to ask colleagues for help and support: "[Y]ou don't feel comfortable when you're already – I can say – 31 or 32 and always just asking questions, yes? (…) [Y]ou want to be independent, yes, and so it's always a bit uncomfortable" (IP08: 44).[158]

Less experienced migrant doctors perceived the situation as unbearable. Dr Gregory House remembered: "I always had the impression that I was in the middle of the way, and that I bother everyone, and that I can't help. That was, that was bad for me. I was practically a burden for a couple of months here. And I felt that" (IP07: 87).[159]

He perceived this fact as particularly severe knowing that he got employed in order to meet the shortage of physicians, and to de-burden his colleagues.

---

156 „Also, es ist meine Probleme, dass ich Überstunden machen soll, weil ich zu viel, also nicht, also… Weil ich weniger Erfahrung habe" (IP04: 133).

157 „[S]onst schreibe ich jetzt ein, einen Entlassungsbrief für drei bis fünf Minuten und damals habe ich 30 Minuten gebraucht. Und das geht jetzt nicht, dass ich für 10 Leute dann sechs, fünf, sechs Stunden hier @sitze, oder für mehr@, das habe ich dann zu Hause gemacht, ne" (IP20: 32).

158 „[M]an fühlt sich nicht wohl, wenn man schon - ich kann sagen - 31 oder 32 ist und immer einfach Fragen stellt, ja? (…) [M]an möchte selbständig sein, ja? Und das ist immer ein bisschen unkomfortabel, ja?" (IP08: 44).

159 „[I]ch hatte immer den Eindruck, dass ich in der Mitte des Weges bin und dass ich alle störe und dass ich nicht helfen kann. Das war, das war schlimm für mich. Ich war praktisch eine Belastung ein paar Monate hier. Und ich hab das gespürt" (IP07: 87).

Accordingly, he felt very uncomfortable with his inability to work independently.

'I'm ashamed' that's what I thought, because I couldn't speak the language so well. And because I noticed how the others had to be so patient with me (…). Luckily I always had to ask just once. But as a disadvantage, I had to ask every damn thing, with every damn thing I had to ask something. Starting with the graphs to medical things, "How shall I do this, or that or that?" And that took, well that took time (IP07: 85).[160]

Although Dr House showed concern about his colleagues' patience, by stressing the fact that he had to ask just once implying that he learnt faster than others, and thus emphasising his own cognitive abilities, he revealed that his discomfort was not mainly about his colleagues' expectations, but referred to his own self-esteem.

Meeting the colleagues' expectations

Nevertheless, migrant physicians were also aware of the expectations their colleagues had towards them. Due to severe staff shortages, the work load for the individual was very big, as Dr Lea Peters stated: "[W]hen I arrived, the others already expected that I would start to do shifts and to really work as soon as possible" (IP10: 40).[161]

Asked whether she had felt under a lot of pressure, she was ambiguous, but argued that in this way she was able to more rapidly become productive.

Well, it was difficult. But well, it's ok. That way I learnt fast and I think that's better than − I don't know − half a year only being there and doing nothing, that's more difficult. Well, it was no big pressure. Although, this period wasn't easy (IP10: 42).[162]

Her comment that being under pressure to find one's way was better than being there without doing anything bears two different notions. First of all, it again reveals a sense of self-esteem which is bound to a professional value of self-sufficiency and independence. She wanted to be helpful and of high value to the team. At the same time, it also includes the expectations of her colleagues who were under a lot of stress and expected her to take work off their hands.

---

160 „‚Ich schäme mich' das hab ich, daran hab ich gedacht. Weil ich die Sprache nicht so gut konnte. Und weil ich hab gemerkt, wie die anderen so viel Geduld mit mir haben müssen (…). [B]ei mir war das immer so, ich musste glücklicherweise nur einmal fragen, aber als Nachteil, ich musste jedes Scheißding, bei jedem Scheißding was fragen. Von den Kurven bis zu medizinischen Sachen, wie soll ich das machen, oder das machen oder das machen und das hat Zeit, also das hat Zeit gedauert" (IP07: 85).

161 „[A]ls ich gekommen bin haben die schon alle erwartet, dass ich so schnell wie möglich anfange Dienste zu machen und so richtig zu arbeiten" (IP10: 40).

162 „Naja es war schwierig. Aber naja ist gut, dann habe ich es schnell gelernt und… @(.)@ Ich denke ist besser als, weiß ich nicht, ein halbes Jahr nur ja, da, da sein und nix zu machen ist schwerer. Naja, es, es war kein großer Druck. Obwohl es, obwohl diese Zeit damals nicht einfach war, ja" (IP10: 42).

Dr Christa Brinkmann even felt that she was under special observation due to her status as a migrant doctor. She had the impression that she was not really welcome in the hospital and thus wanted to avoid being an additional burden to her colleagues.

[O]f course we foreigners were not welcomed with open arms by everyone here. (…) [A]nd then I was a bit worried that the other colleagues don't have so much time to listen to what I'm saying. Then it's a bit, yes, difficult @(.)@ (IP01: 26).[163]

Her statement implies that her colleagues had treated her impatiently before, and she was afraid of giving them cause for repeated conflicts.

Also Dr Matteo Moreau argued along these lines when being asked about why he was ready to work many extra hours. He stated: "[B]ehind this is simply that you prove yourself, that you show, 'I can do it'. Firstly. And secondly, that you don't give any reason for criticism" (IP20: 113).[164] Hence, apart from wanting to prove themselves for their own self-esteem, migrant physicians also wanted to show their capability to their colleagues to not be vulnerable for not doing their job, which again implies that he perceived a certain pressure in this respect.

Increased self-esteem over time

The high appreciation of the value of autonomy and its relevance for the respondents' professional self-concept was further emphasised by migrant physicians' statements about how they felt when this phase was finally over, and they managed to accomplish their work and tasks self-sufficiently. In these accounts, again, the independence from the colleagues played a major role. This was the case for Dr Meredith Grey who reflected: "I found myself. I could work faster. I knew what I had to do and so on, how the procedures are. I was totally independent of the others and that was also very important to me" (IP14: 251).[165]

Dr Gregory House felt rewarded when he was finally in the position to help others (IP07: 285). After having gained this independence, he had finally managed to meet his own expectations, and to successfully transfer his professional self-concept to the German work environment. "I had the impression, now I made it, now I finally am a doctor" (IP07: 105).[166] With regard to the

---

163   „[N]atürlich wir Ausländer hier sind nicht so mit offene Hände von jede gewartet so. (…) [U]nd dann ich bin ein bisschen, ehm, also, ich habe Sorgen, dass eh, die anderen Kollegen haben nicht so viel Zeit, mir zu eh, alles eh, zu, was ich erzähl, ihm zu hören oder so, dann ist ein bisschen, ja schwierig @(.)@" (IP01: 26).

164   „[D]ahinter steckt einfach äh, dass man sich bewährt, dass man zeigt, 'Ich kann es machen'. Erstens. Und zweitens, dass man keinen Grund für ähm, äh, für Kritik dann bekommt" (IP20: 113).

165   „Ich habe mich gefunden. Ich konnte schneller arbeiten. Ich wusste was ich machen soll usw., wie die Abläufe sind. Ich war total unabhängig von den anderen und äh, das war mir auch ganz wichtig" (IP14: 251).

166   „Ich hatte den Eindruck, jetzt habe ich geschafft, jetzt bin ich endlich Arzt" (IP07: 105).

relationship with colleagues and also superiors, Dr Lea Peters felt more secure and self-confident after some time when having found her position in the team.

[I]n the beginning I was very shy @(.)@, and now I can, I mean, if I want something, I simply feel more confident. With the head physician, with the senior physician, if I want something, I can say that directly, I'm no longer shy. I already have my @position@ (IP10: 136).[167]

The same applied to Dr Matteo Moreau who had become more assertive over time. Asked about what had changed for him, he replied: "That now I watch out more for the rights of an assistant physician. Before, as I said, for everything: 'Doesn't matter, now I only have to make sure that I manage to do my work" (IP20: 97).[168] While initially he had tried to please everybody, and to prove himself and his abilities, he now set certain limits, for instance, refusing to work long extra hours and taking over additional tasks and responsibilities.

Continually gaining work experience on-site did not only increase the migrant doctors' standing towards their colleagues, but also their acceptance by patients. Accordingly, Dr Christina Yang explained:

The whole medical experience is different, that changed everything. I can communicate much better with the patients and they can @trust@ me so much more, because I'm more confident and everything, yes, that's become better (IP18: 289).[169]

Therefore, experience helped the respondents to get others' recognition, but also to be able to recognise themselves in their role as a medical doctor.

In sum, drawing on a professional culture that promotes infallibility and self-sufficiency, the migrant physicians suffered from their initial inability to transfer their professional self-concept to the new working environment. The sentiment of incompetence, as well as the perceived lack of clinical autonomy strongly impaired the migrant physicians' self-esteem. In particular, the impression of being a burden to others was emphasised as unbearable. This was additionally triggered by the expectations they felt their colleagues had towards them vis-á-vis the pressing situation on ward. Hence, the migrant doctors identified a mismatch between the requirements towards them as practicing physicians in a German hospital, and their capability to fulfil their tasks on-site. Additionally, the pressing staff situation, which they initially perceived

---

167 „[A]m Anfang war ich sehr schüchtern @(.)@ und äh, jetzt äh, kann ich meine, also wenn ich was will und äh, ich fühle mich einfach sicherer. Mit dem Chefarzt, mit dem Oberarzt, wenn ich was will, dann kann ich das gleich sagen ob ich, ich bin nicht mehr schüchtern. Ich habe schon meine @Position@" (IP10: 136).

168 „Dass ich jetzt äh, mehr auf die Rechte des Assistenzarztes achte. Also vorher wie gesagt, für alles, „Ja ist egal, ich muss jetzt nur da zusehen, dass, dass ich meine Arbeit schaffe"" (IP20: 97).

169 „[D]ie ganze medizinische Erfahrung ist anders und ähm, das hat geändert alles. Also ich kann besser mit den Patienten unterhalten und die können mich deutlich mehr @vertrauen@. Weil ich bin sicherer und alle und ja, das ist besser geworden" (IP18: 289).

as enabling their migration, was now perceived as complicating their professional incorporation since it triggered high expectations towards them on the part of their colleagues.

Nevertheless, the migrant doctors did not request additional support and some even refused to ask their German (-trained) colleagues for help. Instead, they put up with the lack of incorporation measures provided on the part of the hospital administration, and the expectation towards them to immediately blend in and take over full responsibility. Relatedly, they were eager to solve occurring problems and difficulties themselves. Thus, they wanted to prove to themselves and others that they are capable of their position. This coping strategy was motivated by the entrenched professional norm of clinical autonomy that they identified with, the high expectations on the part of their colleagues, as well as with the wish to legitimise their migration. Since they primarily migrated for career development, the inability to fulfil this endeavour would have questioned the entire undertaking and exacerbated the notion of failure. By quickly adjusting themselves to the local standards by their own means, they eventually overcame this uncertainty.

6.2.5 Entering inter-professional struggles – the "migrant doctor-nurse game"

Most of the migrant physicians stated to have a good relationship to other physicians on ward and appreciated the cooperation and encouragement. For instance, Dr Matteo Moreau was pleased about the patience his colleagues had had with him stating that they "simply showed understanding for me being slower and not managing everything that well. Yes, that's what it was like" (IP20: 30).[170] This also applied to Dr Leyla Sherbaz who perceived her team on ward as very supportive. "That was very supportive, like, 'Don't panic. Keep going, that'll slowly become better.' Yes, in this respect it was very, very nice.'" (IP24: 93).[171] However, in most cases, this supportive atmosphere did not apply to the relationship the migrant physicians had with the nurses onsite.

The relationship between nurses and doctors is shaped by a strict hierarchy (Freidson, 1970, p. 52f.), differing courses of education, as well as a gendered division of labour, and stereotypical gender roles with predominantly women as nurses doing the care work (Sander, 2009; Sweet & Norman, 1995), although more women are becoming physicians, and male nurses are no longer

---

170 „[E]infach Verständnis gezeigt haben, dass ich jetzt langsamer bin und dass ich nicht alles so gut schaffe, ähm, ja genau, das war so" (IP20: 30).

171 „Das war eher so (3) Unterstützung, ja und so, alles so, 'Keine Panik. Weitermachen, das wird langsam besser.' Ja, so von daher war das hier sehr, sehr nett" (IP24: 93).

uncommon. In his prominent study "The doctor-nurse game" Stein (1967) described this special relationship in terms of an implicit agreement on interaction on ward that keeps up appearances of a subservient position of the nurses towards the physicians. In fact, the nurses are expected to take initiative and make recommendations, but have to appear passive at the same time, while the physicians ask for recommendations in the same subtle manner keeping up the notion of omnipotence and omniscience. If either of the parties did not participate and play by the rules, one would not cooperate in the expected manner in following interactions.

However, together with colleagues, Stein revised this observation in 1990 (Stein, Watts, & Howell, 1990). They then stated the unilateral termination of this agreement by the nurses striving for a greater acknowledgement of their work and the nursing profession in general. According to Stein et al., this lead to nurses being more outspoken in their recommendations, challenging physicians on certain decisions, and being more independent in their work, thus contravening the traditional hierarchy. This behaviour was also identified by Hughes (1988), particularly in informal situations when matters had to proceed quickly, and in interaction with young, inexperienced physicians to whom they openly gave recommendations. Additionally, he found that this behaviour on the part of nurses was even amplified when interacting with migrant doctors. More experienced nurses took control over the situation. They rephrased the patients' statements when the doctor had difficulties understanding, and also when the doctors' lacking familiarity with the social and cultural context on-site lead to misunderstandings. They also openly criticised and corrected the migrant physicians, and made fun of mistakes these doctors made, e.g. with formulations on treatment cards. Hughes (1988) explains this behaviour with Everett Hughes' (1945) concept of a "dilemma of status." He refers to a conflict between the migrant doctors' high professional status contradicting a lower status attributed to migrants. This status as migrant is regarded as an auxiliary characteristic that often overshadows social status based on profession. The dilemma further evolves based on the experience-based advantage the nurses have towards the migrant doctors who are unfamiliar with the local language and local habits.

Using Bourdieu's notion of cultural capital (Bourdieu, 1984), this 'dilemma of status' can be captured as symbolic devaluation of formally recognised cultural capital. However, the capital's value can be re-negotiated. To this end, migrants engage in symbolic struggles with those devaluing their capital (Nohl, Schittenhelm, Schmidtke, & Weiß, 2010a). These symbolic struggles can take various forms, and have different outcomes. For the case of the doctor-nurse relationship, Pullon (2008) found that inter-professional trust is based on credibility, i.e. demonstrated competence. Only when proving one's skills and expertise, mutual respect develops and eventually turns into a trustworthy relationship. Through this process, cultural capital that had been symbolically devalued based on characteristics such as the status as migrant, can be again valorised.

Hence, one strategy the migrant physicians employed to cope with the uncertainty caused by the devaluation of their skills was again to quickly adapt to the local work culture using the strategy of *protective action*. However, they also employed the strategy of "certainty construction" (Zinn, 2004) in that they interpreted the situation according to the expectations towards a nurse prevailing in their countries of origin, thus degrading the nurses' responsibilities in order to assure their superior status as medical doctor and restoring certainty.

'Dilemma of status'

The dilemma of status with regard to the relationship between nurses and the migrant doctors as described by Hughes (1988) was also experienced by the migrant physicians under study. Dr Karin Patzelt felt that her missing experience undermined the usual hierarchy between physician and nurse, and lead to a dilemma of status, and thus competition between her and the nurses. Referring to her initial phase on ward, Dr Patzelt reported: "That was a bit difficult, because I know how I was in the beginning, they had more experience than me and then there was no respect between us" (IP25: 142).[172] This lack of respect was expressed by one nurse emphasising that she did not need any instructions from Dr Patzelt. "[S]he said to me: 'OK, I'm working here for 40 years, you don't have to tell me how much anaesthetic to give'" (IP25: 150).[173]

However, in the case of the migrant physicians the dilemma of status was not only based on the nurses' longer clinical experience, but was further amplified by the physicians' migrant status and their language difficulties. Asked for the reasons of her difficult relationship to the nurses, Dr Lea Peters replied: "[B]ecause I'm young and because I'm a [national of CEE country]. Sometimes I think like that. And they've to listen to me @(.)@. Yes, and sometimes when I say something, they don't really want to listen to me" (IP10: 72).[174] Due to these attributes she felt that she did not convey the necessary authority, and nurses did not pay her the respect that would be appropriate according to her position. Additionally, difficulties with the German language gave cause for disrespectful behaviour on the part of the nurses, as Dr Peters further elucidated: "I conducted the anamnesis and I wrote everything down and then she

---

172 „Das war ein bisschen schwierig weil ich weiß es, wie ich bin am Anfang und sie haben mehr Erfahrung als ich und dann war zwischen uns, war, war kein äh Respekt" (IP25: 142).

173 „[S]ie sagt mir: 'OK ich arbeite hier 40 Jahre, Du musst mir nicht sagen wie viel äh, ja Anästhetikum muss ich verabreichen' so" (IP25: 150).

174 „[W]eil ich jung bin und weil ich äh, äh, [Staatsangehörige von moe Land] bin. Manchmal denke ich so. Und sie müssen auf mich hören @(.)@. Ja. Äh, und manchmal wenn ich was sage und sie sind äh, dann wollen sie dann nicht so richtig auf mich hören" (IP10: 72).

read it and she realised that I had made a mistake and then she laughed about it with another nurse" (IP10: 70).[175]

Again, the ability to display competence was not given undermining Dr Peters' position towards the nurses and thus leading to a symbolic devaluation of her cultural capital, i.e. her medical skills and expertise.

Symbolic Struggles

The contradiction between formal recognition and the experience of disrespect from nurses led to symbolic struggles in which positions in the hierarchy were negotiated. These disputes were carried out between nurses and migrant physicians in different situations. The nurses took advantage of the physicians, for example, by refusing to show consideration for the migrant doctors' level of German language proficiency, as pointed out by Dr Susan Lewis: "[T]hey know that I don't understand the [regional] dialect and have only standard German, but insist on talking in a [regional] dialect @(.)@" (IP04: 75).[176] The nurses deliberately excluded her emphasising their presumed greater rights on-site, as well as their expectations of her to adapt to the local circumstances. They purposefully did not rectify misunderstandings that they observed, as Dr Kathrin Globisch felt: "Already a couple of times we had the problem that I say, this and that shall be done. They didn't realise, they didn't ask about it, and then it's my fault that it didn't get done, yes" (IP05: 52).[177] She had the impression that the nurses did not make enough effort to support her in order to ensure a smooth flow of work, but more or less deliberately let her fail in order to prove her incapability. Such behaviour was also observed by Dr Doug Ross who, now being a more experienced physician, commented on the way some nurses treated less experienced junior doctors, irrespective of national origin.

[S]ome are, well like salt in the wound. (…) You've difficulties and you're agonizing and then someone comes and says, "Euheuheuh, that didn't work out" or, "That's not good", and makes you even more insecure and they like doing that (IP17: 114/116).[178]

---

175 „[I]ch habe Anamnese gemacht und ich habe das äh, alles aufgeschrieben und dann hat sie das gelesen und sie hat es äh, sie hat bemerkt, dass ich da einen Fehler gemacht habe, ja und dann hat sie mit der anderen Schwester gela-, darüber gelacht" (IP10: 70).

176 „[D]ie wissen, dass ich keinen [regionalen] Dialekt wissen und nur Hochdeutsch gehört habe, aber sie wollen nur [regionalen Dialekt] sprechen @(.)@" (IP04: 75).

177 „Es gab schon ein paar Mal das Problem, dass ich sag, das und das soll gemacht werden. Sie haben das nicht mitgekriegt, sie hatten das nicht nachgefragt und dann bin ich schuld, dass das nicht gemacht wurde, ja" (IP05: 52).

178 „[M]anche sind, ra wie Salz auf, auf der Wunde. (…) Du hast Schwierigkeiten und qualst Dich und dann kommt einer und sagt, ‚Böböbö', was hat nicht geklappt' oder, ‚Das ist nicht gut' oder, und dann macht Dich noch unsicherer und, und das ist, das machen die gerne" (IP17: 114/116).

However, not all of the respondents shared the same experience. Dr Gregory House, for example, stated that he had learnt a lot from experienced nurses and also received a lot of support. "[S]ome of them realise when you're insecure and they step in and they talk to the patient a bit and they calm him and well, 'Don't we want to give that?' and such thing" (IP07: 160).[179]

Hence, just as described by Stein (1967) in "The doctor-nurse game", the nurses took control over the situation, and subtly guided the doctor in his next steps. Corresponding to Pullon's (2008) findings that inter-professional trust between nurses and doctors is based on credibility, Dr Karin Patzelt discovered that in order to achieve the nurses' respect and thus receive their help and support, she had to prove her capability. After major difficulties and many conflicts with the nurses in the initial phase of her employment, she got along with them much better. "I showed a bit that I can do it and I'm not so stupid and OK, I know in the beginning my German wasn't good, but I'm not stupid @(.)@. That's not the same" (IP25: 144).[180]

Thus, mutual respect can develop and eventually turn into a trustworthy relationship. Additionally, this corresponds to the perception stated earlier by respondents that they had to prove themselves and their capability on-site. Thus, migrant doctors were given the chance to gain the nurses' favour and goodwill.

Interfering with the migrant physicians' responsibilities

The struggle over jurisdiction is one of the most prominently discussed topics with regard to professions (Abbott, 1988). While this is mostly done on a structural level, it also played a role in the everyday routine of the migrant physicians under study. As depicted above, migrant physicians struggled with the inability to appear competent, and thus experienced a lack of respect and subordination on the part of nurses. Hence, respondents perceived some nurses to occasionally exceed their competences and jurisdiction by not accepting, and indeed interfering with, decisions taken by the migrant doctors. Drawing on their vast clinical experience, nurses often had an experience-based advantage towards the migrant physicians. However, sometimes their "knowing-better" was perceived as patronising and invasive.

This was experienced, for instance, by Dr Julia Berger when doing shifts in the intensive care unit. She felt that she was treated condescendingly by the nurses and had the impression that they did not trust her to make the right decision. Thus, she did not feel acknowledgement for her medical expertise and

---

179 „[M]anche von denen merken schon, wenn du unsicher bist und die springen dann ein und die sprechen mit den Patienten noch ein bisschen und die beruhigen den und naja, ‚Wollen wir nicht das geben?' und so ein Ding" (IP07: 160).

180 „[I]ch habe ein bisschen gezeigt, dass ich kann das machen und ich bin nicht so dumm und OK, ich weiß am Anfang ich kann nicht so gut Deutsch sprechen, aber ich bin nicht dumm @(.)@ Das ist nicht das gleiche" (IP25: 144).

skills. "'I've respect for them working up there at the intensive care unit, and knowing so much about the intensive care unit and therapy. But maybe they should also recognise the fact that some things we maybe know better" (IP29: 89).[181]

Additionally, interviewees identified certain inflexibility on the part of the nurses with regard to certain medical decisions. This happened particularly when migrant doctors proceeded in a way that did not match the usual or traditional way taken by German (-trained) physicians on-site, and thus deviated from the common routine, as was reported by Dr Susan Lewis with regard to the medication and dosages she prescribed for patients.

[W]e've already learnt that sometimes we can give one or the other drug having the same effect, and when I then decide for one, but other physicians would have decided for the other, and the nurse sees that I give the one, while the other medical specialists would have given the other, they don't like it. Or sometimes I give a different dosage than is common to do here, and she is annoyed with that (IP04: 77).[182]

Hence, she emphasised the lead in expertise she had towards the nurses and stressed that different procedures can have the same effect. In the same vein, namely through distinction, Dr Martin Stein who was close to finishing residency at the time of the interview entered these inter-professional struggles. He argued: "[T]he difference between physicians and nurses is that the nurses do everything according to the standard, or they don't do it. The physicians can deviate from the standard if they know when and for what reason" (IP08: 86).[183]

By stressing his expertise and distancing himself from the nurses, he fought back, thus engaging in the struggle and defending his higher position in the hierarchy. He further explained how to convince the nurses to follow his instructions. "Then of course you've to prove that everything is good, that's wanted. Then the nurses do it, yes?" (ibid.).[184] Hence again, proving oneself and one's own knowledge and competence to the nurses was suggested as solving the problem.

---

181 „[I]ch habe Respekt dafür, dass sie dort oben auf Intensiv arbeiten, und, und so viel auch wissen über Intensivstation oder Therapie. Aber vielleicht sollten sie auch nachdenken, dass manche Sachen wissen vielleicht wir besser" (IP29: 89).

182 „[W]ir wissen schon, dass vielleicht kann diese geben und diese auch und wenn ich dann entscheide, ,Ok, ich gebe diese', aber die anderen Ärzte die andere und die Krankenschwester sehen nur, dass ich geb diese und nicht diese und die anderen Fachärzte geben nur die andere und es gefällt ihnen nicht. Oder ich gebe nicht zweimal oder dreimal und wir machen es nicht so und sie ärgert sich darüber" (IP04: 77).

183 „[D]er Unterschied zwischen Ärzten und Schwestern ist so, dass die Schwestern machen das nach Standard oder machen das nicht. Die Ärzten kön-, die Ärzte können vom Standard abweichen, wenn sie wissen wann und auch aus welchem Grund" (IP08: 86).

184 „Dann muss man natürlich nachweisen, das ist alles gut, das ist so gewünscht, dann machen die Schwestern das, ja?" (ibid.).

However, particularly young migrant doctors did not always have the confidence to stand up against the nurses' interference, and to defend their decisions. Due to the fact that they were inexperienced and in an unfamiliar environment, they were themselves insecure and doubtful about their competences. This applied to Dr Miranda Bailey who, based on a patient's explicit wish, prescribed a drug intravenously instead of in the form of a pill, which caused anger on the part of the nurse in charge.

Afterwards a nurse came to me, very angry and she asked me why I did that, because the patient didn't have a temperature. Cause you only give this for fever. I said, 'Yes, I know she doesn't have a temperature, but she wanted it for the pain. She says, 'Why? Then she can swallow it.' @Was all this drama, because I so... I couldn't talk anymore, because I totally blushed and [was] totally flustered@ (IP19: 169).[185]

Being confronted in such a harsh way by a nurse, Dr Bailey did not feel confident enough to insist on her viewpoint and her decision by explaining it with factual arguments. She also did not manage to insist on her jurisdiction and authority as the physician in charge. Instead, she was flustered and upset. Hence again, she failed to represent her competence in a way that received recognition from the nurse.

Nurses' work overload

Apart from disrespect due to a lack of experience and German language proficiency, interviewees also identified the nurses' eagerness to avoid additional work. Therefore, this struggle over competences as manifested in the respondents' accounts additionally reflects the increasing workload of nurses in German hospitals that has been caused by recent severe job cuts due to economic motives (Simon, 2012).

Dr Lea Peters experienced that nurses would not accept the decisions she made in her capacity as a medical doctor. She complained about the nurses' interference with her work and responsibilities when they were displeased with her hospitalising patients who had come to the first-aid station. "[T]he nurses always say, that's also work for the nurses and they don't want that. But it's not their responsibility (…). [W]e've a lot of patients and very few personnel. And that's leading to conflicts" (IP10: 74).[186] Empathising with the nurses' dissatisfaction, she identified their high workload and the additional work the inpatient admission would mean for them. This impression was shared by Dr

185 „Danach kam eine Schwester zu mir, sehr böse und sie hat gefragt, warum hab ich das gemacht, weil sie hat kein Fieber. Weil das gibt man, wenn man hat Fieber. Ich sagte, „Ja ich weiß, sie hat kein Fieber, aber sie wollte das gegen Schmerzen.' Sagt sie, ‚Warum? Dann kann sie das schlucken.' @War so die ganze so Theater, weil ich so... Ich konnte nicht mehr so erzählen, weil ich so total rot und fertig@ [war]" (IP19: 169).

186 „[D]ie Schwestern meinen immer, äh, das ist auch die Arbeit für die Schwester und sie wollen das nicht. Aber sie sind dafür nicht verantwortlich (…) [W]ir haben sehr viele Patienten und sehr wenig Personal. Und das, das macht Konflikte bei uns" (IP10: 74).

Susan Lewis. She also felt that the frequent dissatisfaction and frustration of the nurses with migrant physicians was triggered by mistakes migrant physicians made that in consequence collaterally burdened the nurses. "[T]hey don't like these many, many corrections. And they shall work with this thing and it's more work for them, too. And that's why, I think" (IP04: 79).[187]

Accordingly, the migrant physicians had the impression that the nurses perceived them as an additional strain contributing to their overstress. According to Dr Martin Stein, this complementarily explains their impatience. "[T]hey don't have so much patience regarding language with us, they want a quick response, 'Yes. No', but not every decision can be made immediately. So, if there's a lack of time, it's a bit more difficult" (IP08: 84).[188] In the perception of the migrant doctors, the resulting stress significantly strained the working atmosphere on ward, as Dr Lea Peters stated. "[Y]ou've to do everything very fast, and there's also lots to do, and of course when everybody is busy and doesn't have time, that's not really good for the work atmosphere" (IP10: 54).[189]

Degradation of nurses' tasks as a coping strategy

As mentioned above (ch. 5.2.3), there are differences in the jurisdiction of medical doctors and nurses between the physicians' countries of origin and Germany. Tasks such as taking blood samples, establishing vascular access, and putting bandages on patients are conducted by the nurses in most of the home countries of the migrant physicians. However, in Germany these tasks are the responsibility of doctors. Although the migrant doctors adapted to the local task division in the daily routine, they use the fact that in their countries these tasks are seen as minor, and the tasks that nurses in Germany are responsible for ancillary activity, as a strategy to fight back. Thus, they distanced themselves from the nurses in the German hospital by devaluing the nurses' competences. To this end, they interpreted the situation according to the professional order in their countries of origin, thus assuring themselves of their professional identity and restoring certainty.

Commenting on the fact that in German hospitals physicians are in charge for taking blood samples, Dr Miranda Bailey expresses the absurdity she perceives when imagining this task division in relation to the medical profession in her home country. "[I]n [my home country] this is only done by the nurses.

---

187 „[D]iese viele, viele Korrigation eh gefällt ihnen nicht. Und sie sollen mit diese Ding arbeiten und es ist eh, eh mehr Arbeit für sie auch. Und deshalb glaube ich" (IP04: 79).

188 „[S]ie haben nicht so viel Zeit mit Sprache mit uns, sie wollen schnell eine Antwort, 'Ja-nein.', und eh nicht jede Entscheidung kann man sofort treffen. So, wenn Zeit fehlt ist schon etwas schwieriger" (IP08: 84).

189 „[M]an muss alles so schnell machen und ähm, und man hat auch viel äh, zu machen und das ist, das ist natürlich für die, das Arbeitsklima nicht so richtig, wenn alle so beschäftigt sind, äh, und keine Zeit haben und dann ist das nicht so gut" (IP10: 54).

The physicians, @they don't do that@" (IP19: 105).[190] Her amusement when saying this additionally reveals that she associates this task with a lower status, and that in her home country this is regarded as a lower task not worthy to be completed by physicians.

In the same vein, Dr Niklas Ahrend was unhappy with that situation.

At a rough estimate, that's one and a half, two hours work in the mornings. Yes. Maybe one and a half in which (3) we don't have to do that. Yes? Then we can take care of our own stuff, well, of our own in quote. We've regarded that only as the nurses' responsibility (IP21: 79).[191]

Referring to these tasks as "only" a nurse's job he expressed a derogatory attitude towards this work, and the perception of himself as being overqualified for having to take care of it. This disdain of the nurses' responsibilities, again, points to difficulties in the transfer of the physicians' professional self-concept due to differing professional orders between the country of origin and the host country. Dr Matteo Moreau further stressed this impression by his statement that, "[H]ere the nurses only want to distribute trays with food and that's almost where the task of a nurse ends @yes@, the physician has to do the rest (IP20: 10).[192]

This statement reflects the physicians' strategy in the symbolic struggle with the nurses. The degradation and devaluation of the nurses' tasks by reducing them to the distribution of food and medication reveals a lack of appreciation and recognition for the nurses by the migrant physicians. At the same time they distance themselves from the nurses, thus strengthening their own position. In this way, the migrant physicians respond to the questioning of their abilities which poses a threat to their professional identity, thus reconstructing certainty.

In sum, the relationship between nurses and physicians is traditionally tense due to a struggle over jurisdiction and their hierarchical relationship. The latter is usually reversed for young junior physicians, since they initially lack practical work experience. This results in a 'dilemma of status' (E. C. Hughes, 1945) between the two groups. In most cases, this 'dilemma of status' is amplified for the migrant physicians due to several auxiliary characteristics that are used to devalue their position and blur the actual hierarchy. The nurses' work-overload, as well as differences in the doctor-nurse relationship between

---

190 „[I]n [meinem Heimatland], das machen nur die Schwestern und die Ärzte, @die machen das nicht so@" (IP19: 105).

191 „Das sind ähm, ja, grob geschätzt eineinhalb, zwei Stunden Arbeit morgens. Ja. Vielleicht eineinhalb, ähm, wo mi-, wo wir (3) wo wir das nicht machen mussten. Ja? Da könnten wir uns um unsere Sachen, also um unsere in Anführungsstrichen Sachen kümmern. Ähm, wir haben das, nur als so als, als äh, Schwestertätigkeit gesehen" (IP21: 79).

192 „[H]ier wollen die Schwestern nur Tabletten mit Essen verteilen und, somit endet fast die Aufgabe einer Schwester @ja@, da muss der Arzt alles Weitere machen" (IP20: 10).

the medical systems the respondents were socialised in and the German medical system, was identified as additional aspects triggering tensions. The migrant physicians perceived these difficulties as an additional uncertainty, which they coped with by actively adjusting themselves to the local work environment and mentally distancing themselves from the nurses.

6.2.6 Coping with prejudice and discrimination – rationalising symbolic exclusion

Apart from difficulties migrant physicians had with transferring their professional ideal due to problems with their self-concept and with their recognition in their capacity as doctors by others, they also experienced symbolic exclusion. Although most of the respondents stressed their positive encounters with friendly and forbearing patients (e.g. IP01: 90; IP02: 114; IP24: 77; IP29: 99), two interviewees reported to have encountered open racism. Dr Elena Eichhorn experienced the distribution of flyers to local citizens' houses by nurses campaigning against the increasing number of migrant employees at the local hospital (IP09: 58ff.), and Dr Gregory House was exposed to patients complaining about migrant physicians to a nurse, and singing a Nazi-song in his presence (IP07: 170ff.). In other cases, the interviewees could only assume that the respective behaviour of the other party was triggered by the doctor's national origin. They felt that German language deficits and presumed inexperience were employed as a pretext for unequal treatment and exclusion, both by colleagues, nurses, and patients, as well as the migrant doctors themselves. Again, this symbolic devaluation of their cultural capital was perceived as a threat to their status as physicians, since it questioned their professional competence (cp. Bernstein, 2000). Given that they came to develop precisely this competence, the perceived discrimination additionally delegitimised their migration.

In order to cope with this devaluation and de-legitimisation, the migrant physicians again used the strategy of *certainty construction* (Zinn, 2004). They tended to reinterpret these incidences by rationalising them. Rationalisation is, according to Ullah (2010), "the justification of an action performed" and is employed when individuals "feel the need to construct a logical reason for an action of which" they morally do not approve (ibid., 22). In this respect, rationalisation also functions as a defence mechanism against an affront reducing "awareness of the existence of a conflict and its extent and ramifications" (Parsons & Shils, 1967, p. 174). Hence, by rationalising incidences of discrimination, some CEE migrant doctors reinterpreted the situation so that it did not pose a threat to their professional self-concept as well as their migration decision.

As discussed above, migrant physicians were not recognised on the part of nurses to the same extent as German (-trained) physicians, not only due to language deficits and their lack of experience, but also based on their status as migrants. In a similar way, for some the recognition in their capacity as a physician was undermined by the fact that they had not completed medical studies in Germany, but in another country. This was the perception of Dr Elias Bähr, a young physician who had already gained work experience in his home country as well as in another Western EU member state. He recalled an encounter with a nurse when starting his first night shift in the intensive care unit of the German hospital he worked at.

[H]e said, (…) "You're not allowed to do shifts here." – "What do you mean?" – "You've no clue about these things." I was so surprised. Well, for two years I had worked at the cardiology intensive care unit @(.)@, and this nurse comes saying, "You're not allowed to do shifts. You've no clue" (IP28: 128).[193]

Hence, without knowing him, the nurse did not trust Dr Bähr to be able to manage the night shift in the intensive care unit. He himself assumed that the reason for the mistrust might be the fact that the nurse was suspicious as he did not know about the curriculum of medical studies in Dr Bähr's home country, or simply because he regarded him as a beginner (ibid.).

Dr Julia Berger had similar experiences. In her initial phase at the German hospital, German (-trained) junior physicians refused to help her out when she was insecure about certain issues and needed help and advice.

[T]hey always said that we should always ask the senior physician about therapy or something, because they, they don't want [to explain to us], since then it would be their responsibility. So we'd have to discuss this with the senior physician (IP29: 83).[194]

Again, her colleagues did not trust her professional knowledge and skills. Stating concern for being blamed for mistakes the migrant doctor might make reveals the extent of their mistrust in her capability and medical competence. It additionally involves an open offence. Referring her to the senior physician who is usually only consulted with major issues when colleagues of the same position cannot help, they refused to work with her and thus excluded her from the usual collaboration among colleagues on ward. In a similar vein, the cooperation with her German (-trained) colleagues was difficult for Dr Lea Peters, too. Without directly saying so, she implied that they were reluctant in helping

---

193 „[E]r hat gesagt, (…) ‚Du darfst hier gar keinen Dienst machen.' – ‚Wie meinst Du das?' – ‚Du hast gar keine Ahnung über die Dinge.' Ich war so überrascht. Also ich habe zwei Jahre in, also auf Kardiologie-Intensivstation gearbeitet @(.)@ und dieser Pfleger kommt, ich, ich wusste nicht wer er ist eigentlich nicht, (…) und äh hat gesagt, ‚Du darfst keinen Dienst machen. Du hast gar keine Ahnung'" (IP28: 128).

194 „[S]ie sagten immer, wenn sie etwas jetzt sagen, wegen Therapie oder etwas, wir sollen immer den Oberarzt fragen, weil sie, sie möchten das nicht [uns erklären], weil das ist dann ihre Verantwortung, und wir müssen das mit dem Oberarzt besprechen" (IP29: 83).

her out. Therefore, she chose to approach compatriots with questions instead, even if they were not working on the same ward.

In my department, they're all German, but on cardiology or radiology, so when I've a problem then I can always, yes, call the radiologists and cardiologists and they're so, always so helpful, because ehm, they're also [from my home country]. Ehm, and the staff on my ward there are, ehm, that's good, but it @could be better@ (IP10: 50).[195]

Another form of symbolic exclusion and refusal of cooperation was expressed by patients who did not want to be treated by migrant doctors. This was experienced by Dr Gregory House who described such a situation with a patient as follows: "He talks to you, but he talks in a condescending way, as if anyhow you wouldn't have a clue. And he is waiting anyway for the head physician, because anyway you're the stupid foreign physician who's only doing the blood sample" (IP07: 174).[196]

Asking for a more experienced physician was determined as a common strategy employed by patients in order to avoid being treated by a migrant doctor. In some cases patients did not want to show their distrust so openly. "[T]hey all pay attention not to say that because I'm a foreigner I'm incompetent. (…) But sometimes they go behind my back and ask another physician, 'Is that really like that?'" (IP20: 89).[197] Hence, patients secretly assured themselves of the accuracy of the migrant physician's diagnosis, thus revealing their suspicion of the migrant doctor's competence.

Others again expressed their rejection, and the wish to not be treated by a migrant doctor more openly. However, they referred to the migrant physician's German language deficits as triggering this preference, thus using it as pretext for evading treatment by this doctor. Again, this was depicted by Dr Gregory House. "Some, in rare cases, express themselves very clearly, 'I don't believe that you understand me' and so on, and head off" (IP07: 174).[198] This experience was shared by Dr Theresa Koshka. "There was just once this woman, I tried to talk to her and she told me that she can't understand me and she doesn't want to hear me [again]" (IP30: 80).[199] The patient clearly refused to be treated

---

195 „[B]ei mir auf der Abteilung nicht, äh, bei mir sind alle Deutschen, aber auf der Kardiologie oder auf der Radiologie also wenn ich ein Problem habe, dann kann ich immer, ja, Radiologen oder Kardiologen anrufen und die sind so, immer so hilfsbereit, weil naja, die sind auch [aus meinem Heimatland]. Ähm, und der Mitarbeiter bei uns auf der Station es gibt, äh, es ist schon gut, aber es @könnte besser sein@" (IP10: 50).

196 „Er spricht mit dir, aber er spricht nur von oben so, als ob du sowieso keine Ahnung hättest. Und er wartet sowieso auf den Chefarzt, weil du sowieso der dumme ausländische Arzt bist, der nur die Blutentnahme macht" (IP07: 174).

197 „[D]ie passen schon alle auf, dass sie nicht sagen, dass ich, da weil ich Ausländer bin, bin ich inkompetent. (…) Ähm, aber manchmal gehen jetzt hinter meinem Rücken und fragen dann bei einem anderen Arzt, ‚Ist das tatsächlich so?'" (IP20: 89).

198 „Manche, in seltenen Fällen, äußern sich klar und deutlich, ‚Ich glaube nicht, dass du mich verstehst' usw. und so fort und gehen los" (IP07: 174).

199 „Es gibt nur einmal, es eine Frau, ich versuchte mit sie zu sprechen und sie hat mir gesagt, sie kann mich nicht verstehen, verstanden und sie möchte nicht [noch] einmal mich hören" (IP30: 80).

by her. Despite the previously discussed mistrust of patients in the doctor's competence vis-á-vis their difficulties with the German language, in these present cases, the migrant physicians perceived the rejection, not as being triggered by a lack of confidence, but in fact being based on their national origin. In response to the experienced symbolic exclusion, migrant physicians often took a very careful and apologetic stance. They were very cautious with the identification of experienced discrimination and exclusion as triggered by their national origin, and tended to rationalise unequal treatment with their lack of experience as well as their German language deficits. Correspondingly, they were rather reluctant to identify discriminatory behaviour of nurses, colleagues, or patients towards them as being triggered by their migrant status. Hence, they were very ambivalent and contradictory in their statements and relativized the respective behaviour, as was the case for Dr Julia Berger trying to explain the behaviour of her German (-trained) colleagues towards her.

[W]ell, could be sometimes because we're foreigners. I, yes. Sometimes. (…) So directly, directly nobody told me so, that I'm a foreigner and therefore, or, or, or (2) yes. Hard to say. (…) I don't know, the Germans are sometimes not so @(.)@ nice with us. Could also be, because we're beginners. Of course, sometimes problems result from that, because, if you don't have so much experience and then you do something wrong, or I don't know. Well, directly I wouldn't @say so@ (IP29: 219/221).[200]

Hence, she did not want to accuse her colleagues of racism, but also could not entirely exclude this suspicion. Finding her lack of experience to be a potential alternate explication for the experienced poor treatment, she found a rational and factual way out of this struggle. A similar pattern was shown by Dr Elena Eichhorn with respect to patients.

[T]here are patients who you can actually never satisfy. They're always dissatisfied. And rarely, that at all, that you can hear, or people say that then, they're searching for arguments and then, yes, ok, well say then "the [foreigner]" or… Rarely, rarely. Actually, I couldn't concretely recall such a case. But at some point, yes, there was something like that, yes. But actually not really (IP09: 76).[201]

Arguing that some patients are notoriously dissatisfied, she tried to divert the attention from a potential discrimination based on her national origin, again

---

200 „[A]lso, könnte sein, manchmal deshalb, weil wir Ausländer sind. Ich, ja. Manchmal. (…) So direkt, direkt habe ich, hat das mir noch niemand gesagt, dass ich, dass ich Ausländer bin und deshalb, oder, oder, oder (2) ja. Schwer zu sagen. (…) Weiß ich nicht, die Deutschen sind, sind manchmal nicht so @(.)@ nett mit uns. Könnte auch deswegen sein, weil wir Anfänger sind. Natürlich, davon gibt es manchmal auch Probleme, weil, wenn man nicht so große Erfahrung hat und dann etwas falsch macht, oder weiß ich nicht. Also, direkt würde ich nich-, @so nicht sagen@. Ja" (IP29: 219/221).

201 „[E]s gibt solche Patienten denen kann man nie eigentlich gut tun. Die sind immer unzufrieden. Und äh, selten, dass es überhaupt, dass man dann hört oder es wird erzählt, dass dann, die das dann, die suchen dann nach Argumenten und dann, ja, gut, also sagen dann also ‚die [Ausländerin]' oder... Selten, selten. Eigentlich ich könnte mich jetzt konkret eigentlich an keinen so Fall erinnern. Aber irgendwann ja, gab's das in der Art, ja. Aber eigentlich nicht so wirklich" (IP09: 76).

finding a rational cause for their behaviour. By playing down these named circumstances, she revealed a certain discomfort with the statement. However, in her case the vagueness did not refer to an uncertainty about the true motivation behind the described demeanour, as in the case of Dr Julia Berger, but to the actual occurrence thereof. A reason for this unease on her part might be embarrassment. This was stated by Dr Gregory House when describing his feelings vis-á-vis experienced discriminatory behaviour towards himself. "[W]hen something like this happens and when you understand the situation, then it's somehow embarrassing" (IP07: 178).[202] This abashment could result from the devaluation of the physicians' cultural capital, and thus of their status as physician. Hence, it again threatened their professional self-concept.

Also in other cases respondents rationalised experienced exclusion with their own shortcomings, such as language deficits and a lack of professional experience. However, they did so to an extent to which they normalised this kind of treatment and thus adopted this position for themselves. This applied to Dr Mark Greene explaining how he felt disadvantaged by his superiors. "During ward round everyone speaks with their German colleagues rather than with me, because it's a bit slower when they talk to me and when you've lots to do, there's no time for that, to say some things twice" (IP03: 60).[203] He justified his exclusion with the time shortage everyone had to deal with and conceived the fact that he got excluded from the discussion and thus, to a certain degree, from his specialist training, as the normal course of events that he had to accept given his level of language proficiency. Dr Susan Lewis underpinned this perceived implicitness: "Well, if we wouldn't be in Germany, but in [my home country] and I had a [native] and an Arab colleague, I'd also talk to the [native] colleague, simply because [it's] easier" (IP04: 60).[204] By putting herself in the other person's position, she further emphasised her understanding for the other's behaviour, stressing its traceability.

This is again amplified by the statement of Dr Christa Brinkmann:

[W]hen there are questions by a nurse, then she asks different colleagues, not me. So, for example, because she's not sure yet whether it's right what I say or not. But that's

---

202 „[W]enn sowas passiert und wenn man die Situation versteht, dann eh, ist sie irgendwie peinlich" (IP07: 178).

203 „Bei der Visite spricht jeder eher mit den deutschen Kollegen als mit mir, weil das ist, es geht ein bisschen langsamer, wenn sie mit mir sprechen und wenn man viel zu tun hat, hat kein Zeit dafür, dass einige Dinge zweimal zu erzählen" (IP03: 60).

204 „Also, wenn wir nicht in Deutschland, sondern in [meinem Heimatland] wären und ich hätte eine [einheimische] und eine arabische Kollegin, ich würde auch mit [einheimische] Kollegin sprechen, weil es einfacher [ist]" (IP04: 60).

also normal. That's nothing, that... Actually, I psychologically prepared for this situation beforehand. Therefore, something like this was not totally unexpected and I wasn't so shocked (IP01: 86).[205]

Hence, Dr Brinkmann did not only identify the nurses' behaviour as normal, but also stated to have expected it. That way, she further increased its presumed naturalness. All three of the respondents thus justified the discriminatory behaviour and exclusion. She further emphasised this by stating that she did not feel that she was in the position to have any demands, hence, distancing herself from the situation by finding a rational explanation. "If I get help here, it's good, but I can't say, 'Well, I'm now expecting someone to help me.' (…) [B]ecause I'm coming to a different country and so I can't tell anyone, someone else is responsible to help me" (IP01: 48/50).[206]

Dr Miranda Bailey did not feel in the position to complain either, for a different reason. After a successful job interview, she was supposed to take up employment in a German hospital as soon as she had received her medical license. While waiting for it, she completed an internship on ward in order to become familiar with the new working environment. However, contrary to a previous agreement, she was provided a contract for a half-time position instead of a full-time position once she received the license. The reasons given for that were insufficient German language skills as well as a lack of experience (IP19: 20). Nevertheless, she was asked to work full time so that she could get further accommodated. Hence, in spite of identifying her German language skills as insufficient, the hospital administration regarded her professional competence as sufficient to work full-time. Although others told Dr Bailey that they did not perceive the given reasons as justified (IP19: 75/81), she did not feel that she was in a position to complain or object.

[T]he head physician talked to me and asked whether I would agree to this and yes, I couldn't say anything else. (…) Yes, because I came to Germany, got my first position and if I would have wanted to say 'no', then, what could I've done? *(IP19: 20/22).[207]*

Dr Bailey was afraid of losing her job. From a later standpoint she rationalised the arrangement: "Actually, that was good for me, because like this I could

---

205 „[W]enn gibt es Fragen, von den Schwestern, dann fragt sie andere Kollegen, nicht mich. So z.B., weil sie noch nicht sicher, ob was ich sage ist richtig und so. Aber das ist auch normal. Das ist nicht etwas, das... Eigentlich ich habe für diese Situation psychisch vorneweg vorbereitet. Deswegen war so etwas nicht ganz unerwartet und ich war nicht so erschrocken" (IP01: 86).

206 „Wenn ich hier Hilfe bekomme, ist gut, aber ich kann nicht sagen, 'Na, ich erwarte jetzt jemanden, mir zu helfen und so.' (…) [W]eil ich komme in andere Land und so ich kann nicht jemand sagen, jemand anderes ist verantwortlich, mir zu helfen" (IP01: 48/50).

207 „[D]er Chefarzt hat mit mir so gesprochen und gefragt, ob ich bin damit so einverstanden und ja. Konnte nichts anderes sagen. (…) Pff, ja weil ich habe, ich bin so in Deutschland gekommen, habe meine erste Stelle bekommen und wenn ja, wenn ich wollte 'nein' sagen, dann, was konnte ich machen?" (IP19: 20/22).

learn a little more and so on. That was good, that was ok" (IP19: 73).[208] Thus, she gained a certain distance to the offense and did not have to admit it. Due to her own insecurity and doubts about her own competence, she did not claim her right to equal treatment, but rationalised the incidence.

In sum, the respondents were hesitant and reluctant to talk about discrimination, and very cautious of accusing others of treating them a certain way based on their national origin. Some of them expressed their suspicion that colleagues and patients did not trust their qualifications. However, mostly the respondents downplayed or rationalised their experiences. This might be due to their own insecurity about the true motivation behind a certain incident. It also reflects their discomfort with such a situation and their attempt to protect themselves from this offence, since it means a devaluation of their cultural capital and their non-recognition in their capacity as a physician. By naming their experiences of symbolic exclusion, they would admit the failure in the transfer of their professional status. Therefore, they tried to circumvent this painful confession by rationalising their experiences and thus protecting their professional identity, again employing the strategy of *certainty construction* (Zinn, 2004) by re-interpreting their initial expectations.

6.3 Balances and future plans

6.3.1 Reflecting upon initial expectations – (mis-)matches of conception and reality

CEE physicians come to Germany with certain expectations. Primarily they hope for a different organisation and conception of the medical profession compared to their home countries. This included an institutional conceptualisation of the medical profession, as well as the role and social standing of physicians, and thus their professional self-concept. Consequently, the "double frame of reference" to both the home and host country as indicated by Nowicka (2012) played a crucial role for the migrant doctors' evaluations, since they compared the circumstances in the different contexts. Satisfaction, expressed as the fulfilment of expectations, varied among the physicians across and even within hospitals. In the following section, migrant doctors' experiences regarding payment and technical equipment, their ambivalent experiences with specialist training and their perceived recognition on the part of superiors, colleagues and patients are presented.

---

208 „Eigentlich war das gut für mich, weil ich konnte so ein bisschen mehr lernen usw. Das war gut, das war in Ordnung" (IP19: 73).

Payment and technical equipment on-site

One significant expectation of CEE physicians with respect to the institutional conceptualisation of the medical profession was better pay. Contrary to Wolanik Boström and Öhlander (2012) findings found for Polish migrant doctors in Sweden, the CEE migrant doctors under study stated that they would earn the equivalent of what German (-trained) physicians in Germany earned. Accordingly, physicians were classified in pay scale groups according to their stage of residency, explained by Dr Christa Brinkmann: "Actually that was clear right from the beginning, there's a structured payment for the first year, for the second... For me it's the same as for everyone else" (IP01: 139).[209]

Particularly, the young junior physicians were satisfied with the amount of money they received, since it enabled them to have a 'normal life' in terms of being able to complete their residency without financial pressure as they had envisioned when making their migration decision. Therefore, the overall amount as such was less crucial to the migrant doctors than the fact that they were able to live off it, as Dr Elias Bähr stated:

There, in my home country, I received 500. But living costs are the same. Only renting an apartment is less expensive, but food is the same. Maybe a little cheaper, more expensive, doesn't matter. But here the salary is much higher. So you can get by. (...) As long as I can learn here, I'm not that interested right now (IP28: 239/241).[210]

This account emphasises the priority of career advancement migrant physicians attribute to their establishment in the German medical field. They perceive this time of training abroad primarily as a status passage in which their training and the training conditions are more salient than, for instance, to make a lot of money. This is stressed by the fact that those migrant physicians who had spent more time in Germany, already finished residency, and entered the next career step, had higher demands in terms of payment. Their perception thereof had over time and with progressing establishment on-site adapted to those of local physicians.[211] Accordingly, when asked about whether he is satisfied with his salary, Dr Niklas Ahrend, already working in Germany for six years, stated: "One shouldn't exaggerate and say 'no'. As a physician you rarely or never become rich, but realistically speaking, yes, it's alright. (...) One would always wish for more, that's obvious. But it's, it's ok" (IP21:

---

209 „Eigentlich das war vom Anfang schon gesagt, gibt es so eine strukturierte Bezahlung in erstem Jahr, in zweitem Jahr... Und wie es für alle, so ist für mich auch" (IP01: 139).

210 „Ich habe dort, [in meinem Heimatland], 500 bekommen. Und das Leben ist das gleiche, nur, nur die Wohnung zu mieten ist äh billiger. Aber Lebensmittel die gleiche. Oder, oder ein bisschen etwas billiger, teurer, egal. Aber, aber das Gehalt hier, also richtig mehr. Also kann man auskommen. (...) [W]enn ich kann hier lernen, interessiert mich nicht jetzt momentan" (IP28: 239/241).

211 On the development of migrants' aspirations over time see Kämpfer (2014).

134/136).[212] Hence, with further career advancement, as well as the advancement in the own life course, priorities and demands of the migrant physicians changed.

Furthermore, the respondents were pleased with the medical possibilities on-site – another aspect that initially motivated their migration decision. For example, Dr Theresa Koshka felt very comfortable being able to treat patients according to their needs without having to consider their financial resources. "Well, for me it's, I don't know, easier to work here. I know what I've to do, and the patient doesn't have to pay extra for that. It's a different world" (IP30: 96).[213] While she particularly enjoyed being able to provide patients with the adequate therapy, Dr Lea Peters stressed the advantages of the technical equipment at her disposal in the German hospital.

[F]or the physician it's important that you don't only make a clinical diagnosis, but that you can also provide a picture, or support the diagnosis with other examinations. That's very important for the certainty of the (physician), and I find that very good here (IP10: 88).[214]

Hence, with regard to their payment and the standard of medical care provided on-site, the migrant physicians were satisfied to have encountered the envisioned circumstances that contributed to their decision to migrate to Germany.

Ambivalences regarding the expected quality of residency

Satisfaction with perceived specialist training

For most of the migrant physicians, their residency and their wish for professional development and progress played the biggest role in their migration motivation. The majority of them felt that their respective expectations were met on-site. Particularly, the training relationship between junior and senior physicians was perceived as very good, and the opportunities for external workshops and trainings were stressed and perceived as beneficial for the own professional progress. Seeking specialist training is another migration motivation. For Dr Mark Greene, a junior physician in his first year, specialist training was

---

212 „Man darf jetzt nicht übertreiben und sagen, 'nein.' Es ist (2), man wird n-, als Arzt sehr selten oder gar nicht reicht, reich, aber ich glaube realistisch gesehen ja, es ist in Ordnung. (…) Man wünscht sich immer mehr, das ist klar. Aber es ist, (2) es ist OK" (IP21: 134/136).

213 „So für mich ist sehr, für mich ist sehr, weiß ich nicht, nicht, ist einfacher hier zu arbeiten. Denn ich kenne das, ich muss das machen und der Patient muss nicht für diese extra bezahlen oder so, ist andere Welt" (IP30: 96).

214 „[D]as ist schon wichtig für den Arzt, dass man nicht nur klinisch Diagnose, die Diagnose stellen muss, sondern kann man auch äh, das Bild geben, oder durch andere Untersuchungen unterstützen, die Diagnose. Und das ist für äh, für die Sicherheit des (Arztes) schon sehr wichtig, ja, und das finde ich sehr gut hier" (IP10: 88).

the main reason to migrate to Germany. He had had high expectations towards the organisation thereof in a German hospital. According to him, these expectations had not been disappointed. He was especially satisfied with the flat hierarchy he perceived exists between junior physicians and their superiors.

I regard as extremely good that here you can approach senior physicians and head physicians directly. That's a taboo in [my home country]. Everyone is very open here, and everyone helps a lot more, and like this you can learn so much faster and much better (IP03: 8).[215]

Likewise, Dr Lea Peters was pleased about the fact that also external advanced training was supported on the part of the hospital and her superior, respectively. "[W]hen I'm interested in something (...) – for example, I wanted to attend this course in Berlin, and the hospital paid for it entirely, and my head physician did not object to let me go for two days" (IP10: 154).[216] Hence, in these cases the migrant physicians' expectations on teacher-student-relationship in the hospital were met. They felt supported in their interest to accumulate and expand their expertise, and thus, in their professional development.

Dissatisfaction with the received specialist training

However, this satisfaction with the training conditions was not shared by all respondents. Six interviewees, both from city and rural hospitals, felt that the current shortage of physicians on-site and the resulting work load for every individual doctor limited them tremendously in their endeavour to acquire encompassing qualifications. They experienced a lack of interest by superiors to provide specialist training due to the struggle of managing daily medical business. In one case, Dr Elias Bähr doubted that it was possible to complete residency within the scheduled time frame.

[H]ow, if you don't learn anything? Well, the senior physicians mostly don't have time to teach us. (...) [O]r we personally don't have time for that. When I return home at 6pm or 7pm, I'm sometimes not in the mood to study anymore (IP28: 343).[217]

Hence, the daily work on ward was given priority over the migrant physicians' training. Dr Lea Peters explained: "You always have to learn so, (...) by the way. You first have to do all the work on the ward, and after you've to, I don't

---

215 „[W]as für mich wahnsinnig gut ist, dass hier kann man z.B. die Oberärzte und Chefärzte direkt ansprechen. In [meinem Heimatland] ist das ein Tabu. Das soll man nicht machen. Hier jeder ist viel offen und jeder hilft viel mehr und man kann so viel schneller und viel besser lernen" (IP03: 8).

216 „[W]enn ich mich für was interessiere (…), wollte ich diese Kurs in Berlin machen und das, das hat das Krankenhaus alles bezahlt und ähm, mein Chefarzt hatte kein Problem damit, dass ich, weiß ich nicht, für zwei Tage nicht da bin" (IP10: 154).

217 „[W]ie, wenn Du lernst gar nichts? Also die Oberärzte haben meistens gar keine Zeit, äh uns zu unterrichten. (…) [O]der wir haben persönlich keine Zeit dafür. Also nach, ich, wenn ich gehe um sechs uhr oder sieben Uhr nach Hause ich habe keine Lust mehr lernen manchmal" (IP28: 343).

know, stay long hours in order to properly learn something" (IP10: 159).[218] Additionally, the staff shortages did not allow the junior physicians to participate in external trainings, as Dr Meredith Grey had experienced with regard to a conference focusing on her specialist field that she wanted to attend in her first year of residency.

I registered, but then I had to change the ward, and I could not attend anymore, because this other ward wasn't catered for, and I had to take care of it alone. And I, for example, did not approve of that. I could have learnt something, but wasn't allowed to because of that. (…). The training doesn't come first. Not for us at least, for the young ones (IP14: 308).[219]

Hence, Dr Grey was not only deprived of the possibility to participate in an event that would have contributed to her professional advancement, but also had to manage an entire ward on her own. This robbed her off the chance to learn from her colleagues, and additionally exceeded her responsibilities at that stage of her career. By mentioning that residency was not of primary concern with regard to young junior physicians, she implied that these in particular were appointed to conduct the routine work instead of being able to pursue their own specialist training. This again reveals a lot about the hierarchy in place. The less experience doctors have, the less importance is attributed to their education.

Dr Julia Berger's impression of her hospital was its focus on maintaining the functionality of the hospital rather than ensure a good and sustainable qualification of its staff. She was also in her first year of residency, and even missed the provision of basic information on the process of specialist training. Consequently, she felt left alone and overwhelmed with planning her residency. Indeed, she lacked the support she needed to get orientation and to successfully complete specialist training.

You've to look up everything online what you really need for specialist-, or the special examination, which medical examinations, how much time you've to spend where. @Here in Germany@, you've to look up these things by yourself, and also residency, you've to choose and organise it, for instance, yourself (IP29: 187).[220]

---

218 „[M]an muss das äh, immer so (…) [n]ebenbei lernen. Also man muss die ganze Stationsarbeit machen und dazu muss man noch in seiner, also weiß ich nicht, muss man länger bleiben um das, um was richtig zu lernen" (IP10: 159).

219 „Ich habe mich auch angemeldet und das hieß es, ich würde Station wechseln. Und ich darf nicht mehr hin, weil diese andere Station nicht versorgt ist und ich muss die Station alleine versorgen. Und das fand ich zum Beispiel nicht gut. Ich hätte etwas lernen können, durfte das aber nicht deswegen. (…) Die Fortbildung kommt nicht erst. Nicht für uns mindestens, für die Jungen" (IP14: 308).

220 „Da muss man alles im Internet nachgucken, was man wirklich für die Weiter- oder für die Fachprüfung was braucht, welche Untersuchungen, und wie viel Zeit wo und ähm, da, ich denke muss man alles selbst nachgucken, @hier in Deutschland@, und, und, die ganze, und die Weiterbildungen auch, muss man selbst aussuchen, und, und dann organisieren zum Beispiel" (IP29: 187).

Ambivalences regarding perceived recognition

Perceived encouragement and recognition

As Bernstein (2000) details, the symbolic recognition of a physician by colleagues and patients has a crucial and positive impact on the physician's wellbeing. Underpinning this finding, the CEE migrant doctors under study gained self-esteem from support and encouragement they received from superiors, colleagues, and patients. The issue of recognition was additionally mentioned as having initially motivated the CEE migrant physicians to leave for Germany, since they perceived a lack of social recognition of medical doctors on the part of patients in their countries of origin.

While others had experienced rejection and mistrust on the part of patients, (see ch. 5.2.6), Dr Mark Greene was pleased with the situation he found in the German hospital; one very different to the one with patients in his home country: "[A]s physician here in Germany, I really like that everyone has... Well, I don't really know how to say this, but people speak to us with (…) respect, yes. And then you feel better in such a position" (IP03: 6/8).[221] Additionally, other respondents appreciated the praise they received from patients (IP05: 92), and perceived the recurrent visits of some patients as a sign of trust (IP17: 176). Patient approval was key in assuring self-esteem and building professional identity of the migrant physicians.

Perceived support and encouragement, which some migrant physicians received from their colleagues and superiors, had the same effect. Thus, they felt recognised for their work on-site as well as in their capacity as junior physicians. This was perceived as such, for instance, by Dr Susan Lewis, who enjoyed that she got professionally challenged by her superior, and felt recognised for her professional performance.

[I]t was a surprise for me that the senior physician wanted me to go to the stroke unit, because there are very difficult patients, and there's more work to do. That's a bigger task than on the normal ward. (…) It's a sign of trust and also a feedback that one is doing something well and on time (IP04: 167).[222]

This was also the case for Dr Meredith Grey who received lauds from her superiors for her performance and positively impacted her work motivation. "I always received positive, not only positive, but also positive feedback and that

---

221   „[H]ier in Deutschland als Arzt finde ich das wirklich sehr schön, dass jede Leute hat eine, na... Ja, das kann ich nicht so gut sagen, aber Leute sprechen mit uns mit eh (…) Respekt, ja. Und, und, und man fühlt sich viel besser in einer solchen Position" (IP03: 6/8).

222   „[E]s war eine Überraschung für mich, dass der Oberarzt wollte, dass ich ins stroke-unit gehe, weil dort schwierigere Patienten geben und eh, mehr zu tun. Und das ist eine größere Aufgabe wie in Normalstation. (…) Und es ist eine Vertrauung auch und eh, auch eine Rückmeldung, dass jemand etwas gut macht und pünktlich macht" (IP04: 167).

was very important. I @felt (valued)@, and then I enjoy working, too" (IP14: 162).[223]

Dr Mark Greene perceived praise on the part of nurses as a particularly important in work motivation; highlighting the often difficult relationship between nurses and migrant doctors. "[T]he nurse once told me: 'Yes, [Dr Greene] can do these things very well', and I've to take that very serious since it was said by a nurse, that's something" (IP03: 90).[224] Hence, being taken seriously, and respected impacted the comfort and confidence of the migrant physicians and contributed to their satisfaction with their own role as a physician. In particular, this speaks to their eagerness to conduct their work self-sufficiently, not being a burden to anyone else. Nonetheless, a positive work climate is appreciated and mutually beneficial for physicians, nurses and other staff, as Dr Michaela Quinn stated:

[W]hen I come to the operating room after a longer time, they, the nurses, say, 'Yes, it's been a long time. Good to have you back' and so on. So I see that they also enjoy working with me. And me too, I enjoy working with them, too. That's always like that, really very good teamwork (IP23: 198).[225]

She perceived the good work climate as very motivating and stimulating for her work routine. It contributed to her well-being in the hospital and made her feel welcome and as part of the team.

Lack of perceived encouragement or recognition

Others again, could not share these positive experiences. Two of the respondents stated to not receive any recognition for their work on the part of their superiors. This was the case for IP28 who missed positive feedback from his head physician. "In [my home country], you always get that from your boss. Like, 'Well done!' and so on. Positive, as well, positive feedback [is] very important. Here, you don't get any" (IP28: 337).[226] Dr Julia Berger highlighted the importance of praise from head physicians: "[Y]ou also don't get a @good word@. For him it's already good if he doesn't say something bad" (IP29:

223 „Ich habe immer positive F-, nicht nur positive, aber auch positive Feedbacks bekommen und das war auch wichtig. Ich habe mich @(wertgeschätzt) gefühlt@ und ich arbeite auch gerne dann" (IP14: 162).

224 „[D]ie Schwester hat mir einmal gesagt, dass, 'Ja, [Dr. Greene] kann sehr gut diese Dinge machen,' und das muss ich sehr ernst nehmen, weil wenn das von einer Schwester kommt, das ist schon was" (IP03: 90).

225 „[W]enn ich äh, nach lang-, längerer Zeit in die OP wieder komme, dann sagen die, sagt die Pflege, "Ja, ich hab Dich lange nicht gesehen. Schön dass Du da bist wieder" und so. Dass, ich sehe, dass die auch Freude daran haben, mit mir zu arbeiten. Und ich bin auch, ich hab auch Freude daran mit Ihnen zu arbeiten. Das ist immer so, wirklich eine sehr gute Teamarbeit" (IP23: 198).

226 „In [meinem Heimatland] Du bekommst das immer vom Chef. Und ,Du hast das gut gemacht' usw. und (3) etwas positiv auch, positiv Feedback sehr wichtig. Es gibt hier keinen" (IP28: 337).

105).[227] Without due recognition, migrant and native physicians alike were likely to feel unwelcome and unmotivated. Additionally, it impaired the transfer of their professional self-concept to Germany.

In sum, in terms of the envisioned structural aspects the migrant physicians hoped to find in the German hospital, the respondents were by and large satisfied. They perceived particularly the hospitals' equipment and resources as favourable for their medical practice. This applied both in terms of fulfilling the medical ethos of providing the best care possible, and in terms of their training being able to learn the handling of modern technical devices. However, when it comes to the organisation of the specialist training, the migrant physicians' evaluations varied. While some were being continuously trained in order to take over responsibilities and build their capacity as doctors, others felt that they primarily served the daily work on ward, working under a subordinate, unwelcoming atmosphere. Consequently, these latter respondents did not perceive recognition or interest in helping complete their residency by their colleagues and superiors

6.3.2 Taking stock – evaluating achievements and losses

In spite of the dissatisfaction with the work atmosphere and the specialist training some of the respondents received in the German hospitals (ch. 6.3.1), almost all of the CEE migrant physicians declared that they would make this migration decision again, and would also recommend to friends and colleagues to do so (e.g. IP01: 176/178; IP07: 329; IP10: 191; IP14: 318; IP28: 355). In their explanation, they indeed consider social migration costs and the experienced indisposition during their initial phase in the German hospitals. However, they weigh these drawbacks against the personal and professional development they made over time, and their favourable financial situation in Germany. In doing so, they again consider two frames of reference, namely, their country of origin and their country of destination. By focussing on the positive features of their migration experience they rationalise the negatively perceived aspects by either assuring that it has been worth the struggle, or that they are better off after their migration to Germany than they would be otherwise. Thus, they cope by legitimising their migration decision, as well as the continuation of their stay in Germany despite dissatisfaction and discomfort with certain aspects.

Reflecting about their migration experience, the CEE physicians emphasised the high costs they accepted in order to come to Germany, which they perceived as an investment that they, hopefully, made for better training and

---

227 „[S]ie bekommen auch @kein gutes Wort@. Also bei ihm ist es schon gut, wenn er nichts Schlimmes sagt" (IP29: 105).

working conditions. Dr Christa Brinkmann, for instance, decided to go to Germany against all odds. For her, the migration decision was connected to adversities regarding her private life and significant pressure due to her being responsible, not only for herself, but also for her family.

I first came here alone. My children followed after a couple of months. My daughter was seven, my son three, four years, and I left my children alone with my husband, and that was difficult, and here it was difficult @yes@. (…) Financially, it was difficult, too. Emotionally difficult, because my parents were a 100% against my decision (IP01: 178/189).[228]

However, those migrating alone also referred to the high migration costs of leaving a familiar home environment. Dr Elias Bähr, for instance, remembered how difficult it was for him to make the decision to migrate. He primarily associated this step with uncertainty, giving up his professionally burdensome, yet stable life not knowing what to expect abroad.

You say, 'Ok, here I've an apartment – doesn't matter. Here I've a car – doesn't matter. Here I've a family – doesn't matter. Here I've a girlfriend – doesn't matter. Here I've two positions, I can live well off those two positions, but whatever, @let's go to Germany@.' I really had cramps in my stomach (IP28: 361).[229]

In their reflections about their migration experience, other respondents particularly stressed the social migration costs in terms of no longer being around family and friends after migration. These social losses and the initial solitude they experienced upon arrival in Germany were major aspects of an initial indisposition they experienced. Accordingly, Dr Meredith Grey, who had migrated to the same city as a friend of hers, still felt alone during the first period of working in Germany as she was missing her boyfriend and her family who she could not visit for six months due to her trial period (IP14: 60). For Dr Niklas Ahrend these losses were still tangible after having been in Germany for seven years. He again stressed the notion of accepting adversities, and thus making an investment in his career. "Of course, you're losing a lot through that. You're not with the parents anymore, you're not with your friends, you no longer have these social things you have at home. They're all sacrificed more or less" (IP21: 224).[230]

228 „[I]ch sollte erst mal hier alleine kommen. Meine Kinder sind danach, nach paar Monaten nach… Meine Tochter war 7 Jahre, mein Sohn 3-4 Jahre und ich habe meine Kinder alleine gelassen mit meinem Mann und so und das war schwierig und hier schwierig und @ja@… (…) Finanziell war auch ganz schwierig. Emotionell schwierig, weil meine Eltern waren 100% gegen meine Entscheidung" (IP01: 178/180).

229 „Du sagst, ‚OK, ich habe hier ein Wohnung egal. Ich habe hier einen Wagen – egal. Ich habe hier eine Familie – egal. Ich habe hier eine Freundin – egal. Ich habe hier zwei Stellen, kann ich damit, kann mit diese zwei Stellen gut leben, aber ach lassen wir, @gehen wir nach Deutschland@.' Ich hatte wirklich Magenkrämpfe" (IP28: 361).

230 „Man verliert natürlich ähm, durch diese Sache sehr viel. Also man ist nicht mehr mit den Eltern, man ist nicht mehr mit den Freunden, man hat nicht mehr dieses soziale ähm, Sachen die man zu Hause hat. Die sind alle geopfert, mehr oder weniger" (IP21: 224).

Whereas Dr Niklas Ahrend did not regret his migration decision, Dr Michaela Quinn who perceived her situation similarly stated that she would not make the same decision again, knowing about the nostalgia she would feel. Although she migrated together with her husband and her daughter, and was satisfied with her professional situation in the German hospital she worked in, she did not feel comfortable in her new living environment. "I think that at the moment homesickness outweighs the great working conditions @(.)@ (IP23: 276).[231]

Others again, who initially did not feel comfortable at their new workplace and who struggled to find their way, particularly emphasised these experiences when looking back. This was the case for Dr Julia Berger, who was already proficient in German when she arrived, but still perceived the process of adjusting and adapting to the new environment as difficult. She expressed these perceived efforts when talking about friends back home in her country of origin as only seeing the positive sides of her working in Germany. "[B]ut they don't see the other side of it, that in the beginning, how much work that was, then moving, to come here, first of all alone, and then struggling here because everything was new, and the language" (IP29: 201).[232]

Dr Gregory House shared this perception. He particularly stressed the indisposition and mental pressure this caused for him. Hence, he mainly referred to the satisfaction of the demands he had put on himself, and thus the transfer of his self-concept which was hampered by him not meeting his own expectations of a physician's role.

The psychological aspect is the problem. Not practically, practically you manage everything as long as you're willing to. But psychologically it's really horrible. And I knew that from the beginning, 'Yes, it's going to be horrible', but I had no idea (IP07: 331).[233]

Despite these emotional and mental difficulties the interviewees stressed, Dr Michaela Quinn was the only respondent who stated that she would not make that migration decision again knowing what to expect. All others stated that they would make the same migration decision again, despite, or explicitly because of, the difficult period in the beginning, wanting their efforts to pay off. Accordingly, the physicians stressed the opportunity for specialist training as such, just as Dr Karin Patzelt who had started residency in a different field in Romania, and then started specialist training anew in her desired field in a Ger-

231   „Ich denke, dass das Heimweh momentan äh, mehr ist als die super Arbeitsbedingungen @(.)@" (IP23: 276).

232   „[A]ber die andere Seite sehen sie nicht, dass, äh am Anfang, wie viel Arbeit das war, und danach auch hier umziehen, hier kommen, erst mal alleine und auch sowieso hier kämpfen wegen, mit alles neu, und Sprache" (IP29: 201).

233   „Psychisch ist das Problem. Nicht praktisch, praktisch schafft man alles, Hauptsache man will. Aber psychisch ist das schrecklich. Und ich wusste das von Anfang an, „Ja, es wird schrecklich sein', aber ich hatte keine Ahnung" (IP07:331).

man hospital (IP25: 256). Additionally, she emphasised her professional development within that time abroad. "I think I've learnt only a small share of what I wanted to learn so far. Until now I've done a lot. More than at home. And lots of practice" (IP25: 375).[234]

Others felt that difficult initial period had been worthwhile as professional perspectives and future career prospects had opened up, such as in the case of Dr Gregory House. "I later talked about it again with the head physician after a year, and he told me that he has plans for me (…), and that was, 'Wow, it was worth it! All the headaches' (IP07: 105).[235] Again, other respondents felt that they had not only developed professionally, but that the adversities and barriers they had faced contributed to their personal development, as Dr Meredith Grey found. "Simply making it on your own is difficult. And yes, it's important to know, that ok, I tried and I made it" (IP14: 316).[236]

Dr Julia Berger who stated to be dissatisfied with the organisation of specialist training and the overall work atmosphere in the German hospital she is working in, admitted that especially in the beginning she sometimes thought about returning home (IP29: 199). Nonetheless, comparing her situation in Germany to the one she left behind in her home country, she found rational reasons for why returning is not an option. Her explanation matches the concept of an envisioned 'normal life' that she and others mentioned as one of the reasons for coming to Germany, and which she would not be able to live in her home country.

[Here] I can learn, have a job and if you're doing well and are industrious, you're not afraid of being dismissed. Well, at home there's such an atmosphere, you don't have a secure position (…). [W]e also achieved such thing that we couldn't achieve at home. For example, that we managed to collect the money for the entire wedding, just the two of us. Actually, we don't need our parents' (IP29: 203).[237]

In general, reflecting about their migration experience, the CEE physicians were positive and stated that they would make the migration decision again. Even the majority of those who again stressed the high migration costs as well as the difficult initial phase in the German hospital stated not to regret this step. They legitimised their migration and the reluctance to return to their home

---

234 „[I]ch glaube, ich habe nur ein wenige Prozent von was ich wollte zu lernen gelernt, schon gelernt über. Bis jetzt habe ich viel gemacht. Mehr als zu Hause. Und viel Praxis" (IP25: 375).

235 „Ich habe darüber nochmal später gesprochen mit dem Chefarzt nach einem Jahr und er hat mir erzählt, dass er Pläne mit mir hat (…) und das war, ‚Wow, das hat sich gelohnt! All diese Kopfschmerzen'" (IP07: 105).

236 „[E]infach alleine klar zu kommen ist schwierig. Und ja (2) ist wichtig zu wissen, OK, ich habe das probiert, ich habe das geschafft" (IP14: 316).

237 „[Hier k]ann ich lernen, man hat eine, eine Arbeit und wenn man, ähm, gut arbeitet und fleißig ist, hat man keine Angst, dass man gekündigt wird. Also zu, zu Hause gibt es auch eine solche Stimmung, man hat keine sichere Arbeitsstelle (…). [W]ir haben auch, ähm, solche Sachen erreicht, was, was wir zu Hause nicht erreichen konnten. Oder zum Beispiel dass, wir haben Geld gesammelt für die ganze Hochzeit, äh, zu zweit, und, äh, brauchen wir eigentlich keine Hilfe von Eltern" (IP29: 203).

countries by emphasising their professional and life opportunities in Germany, thus rationalising their experiences on-site and constructing certainty regarding their migration decision.

6.3.3 Making future plans – impact of the life stage and considered re-migration costs

The majority of the interviewed CEE migrant physicians planned on staying in Germany. While some of the respondents were still open for re-migration, others were determined to not migrate again. The migrants' action orientations in this respect can be partially understood with the help of a life course perspective, focusing among others on "patterns of migrants' biographical mastering of transitions and coordinating of life spheres" (Wingens, De Valk, Windzio, & Aybek, 2011, p. 3). Accordingly, particularly the young migrant doctors conceived of their residency as a status passage, a time in which they gain further qualifications for the transition into the next life stage of work. In their decision of how they planned to approach this next step, they deferred to their private life. Those having a partner and family in Germany planned to remain, whereas those who did not were more likely to re-migrate. From a life course perspective, this correlates with the migrant doctors' biographical age. Having finished training they are on the one hand open to re-migrate since this event marks a transition in their life course that makes migration likely (Kley, 2011). On the other hand, most of the young migrant doctors would be in their thirties after having completed residency – a biographical age in which preferences tend to change towards settling down, and starting a family (Vysotskaya, 2011, p. 101ff.). Having a family, again, increases migration costs and makes re-migration less likely. However, migration costs were also significant in the consideration of the single migrant doctors who were determined to remain in Germany because they feared a loss of professional status gained in German hospitals. Their action orientation to address this feared, repeated uncertainty by staying in Germany represents, again, the coping strategy of *protective action* (Zinn, 2004).

The migrant physicians under study made rather short-term professional plans. As most of them were still in specialist training, their primary aim was to finish residency and become a medical specialist. Hence, they perceived their current situation as a status passage serving to gain qualifications to then progress in career and life. To finish their specialist training, the respondents planned to remain in Germany, at least until having completed residency. However, some of them were rather vague regarding their subsequent planning, such as Dr Karin Patzelt. "I'll certainly stay in Germany for about five years or six, and then I'll pass my special exam, and then I don't know" (IP25: 323).[238]

This openness with regard to the location and the length of stay as well as potential re-migration plans is considered as characteristic for post-accession intra EU migration (Engbersen & Snel, 2013). This vagueness does not only mark the transition from one status passage to another, but at the same time reflects the individualisation of migration patterns enabled, among others, by liberal migration policies in the EU. However, when speculating about what is coming next, respondents who did not have a partner or family stated that their inclination to re-migrate would depend on social rather than professional factors, namely, whether or not they would find a partner in Germany. Dr Patzelt, for instance, saw her future either in Germany or in her home country. "Because of my parents I'd say, I'll return home, but maybe I'll find someone here and get married, @and then I'll stay, I don't know@" (IP25: 381).[239] The same applied to Dr Elias Bähr. "Of course, if I'll find my partner here, then I'll talk to her and if that's the case, I'll stay here. If not, if I don't find anyone, @or not the right one@, then I'll go home or go somewhere else" (IP28: 333).[240]

Again, this shift of priorities in migration decision-making matched the interviewees' life stage. Another explanation could be a generational change that the HR managers and medical directors above referred to as the emergence of the generation Y (see ch. 5.1). The following statement by Dr Gregory House supported this interpretation. "I don't want to be one of those physicians who at the age of 50 are still in the hospital at 8pm doing paper work and seeing patients, because they don't have anything better to do at home" (IP07: 319).[241]

Other respondents were convinced that they would not want to leave Germany again. This applied particularly to migrant physicians who had a partner and children and whose migration decision would not only affect them. Hence again, the respective migrant doctors' life stages influenced their future plans. This was the case, for example, for Dr Doug Ross, who excluded the option to re-migrate to another country in the near future. "That's not going to happen. I can't expect that of my children that they again have to learn a new language. They first have to learn to manage German and [their mother tongue]" (IP17:

---

238 „So fünf Jahre bleibe ich bestimmt in Deutschland und, oder sechs oder dann mache ich meine Fachprüfung, Facharztprüfung und danach ich weiß nicht" (IP25: 323).

239 „[W]egen meine Eltern ich würde sagen ich äh, kehre mich zurück nach Hause, aber vielleicht finde ich hier jemand und ich verheirate mich @und dann bleibe ich, weiß nicht@" (IP25: 381).

240 „Natürlich wenn ich finde mein Partner hier, dann, dann ich spreche mit ihr und, und wenn das so ist, dann ich bleibe hier. Wenn nicht, wenn ich finde niemand, @oder nicht die Richtige@, dann ich gehe nach Hause oder gehe irgendwo hin" (IP28: 333).

241 „[I]ch will nicht einer dieser Ärzte, die mit 50 um acht Uhr abends im Krankenhaus sind und Papier machen und Patienten sehen, weil sie nichts Besseres zu tun Zuhause haben" (IP07: 319).

359).[242] Likewise, the costs were too high for Dr Niklas Ahrend for re-migration, since his wife already once gave up her very good position in their home country to come with him to Germany: "[T]elling her now, 'Let's go to Norway in five years, because there we'll earn 1500 or 2000 Euro more per month.' I can tell almost with certainty, she'll say, 'No. I don't want that'" (IP21: 248).[243]

Nevertheless, also some of the singles were determined to remain in Germany after having finished specialist training. They were afraid of losing again what they had achieved after migrating to Germany. This applied to the investment they had made in terms of efforts to adapt to the new workplace, and thus the position and certainty they had gained on-site, and which they would lose again when having to start anew in another country with yet again a different language and medical system. This was the case for Dr Meredith Grey, who by all means wanted to avoid undertaking the perceived struggle again. "That was so stressful, that was hard. I couldn't sleep at night, I couldn't eat, I lost weight, @I always had nausea, I always was afraid@ to do something wrong. That was really hard. @I don't need that ever again@" (IP14: 330).[244] This fear equally applied to Dr Doug Ross who was concerned about the informal recognition a returning doctor might not be granted in his home country. "[S]tupidly, you'll not come back, let's say, promoted. On the contrary, you've the feeling you're not wanted there anymore. 'Now you're coming from Germany, and what do you want to show me?'" (IP17: 336/338).[245]

In a similar vein, other migrant physicians were afraid of losing something they had acquired by taking up employment in a German hospital. In the case of Dr Christina Yang, this applied to the less hierarchical doctor-patient relationship she got used to while working abroad.

Now my whole attitude has changed. So I can't simply adapt, because in [my home country] physicians are [up] here, and patients are down here at the bottom, and we do

242 „[D]as wird nicht der Fall sein. Ich kann jetzt meinen Kindern nicht zumuten, dass die jetzt noch mal eine neue Sprache lernen, äh, erst muss mal, mit mit dem Deutschen und [ihrer Muttersprache] zurechtkommen" (IP17: 359).

243 „[J]etzt ihr zu sagen, ‚Komm, lass uns nach Norwegen gehen in fünf Jahren, weil wir dort 1500 oder 2000 Euro mehr im Monat verdienen', kann ich fast sicher sagen, da wird sie sagen, ‚Nein. Ich will das nicht'"(IP21: 248).

244 „Das war stressig, das war hart. Ähm, das, ich konnte nachts nicht schlafen, ich konnte nicht essen, ich habe abgenommen @äh, ich hatte immer Übelkeit, ich hatte immer Angst@ etwas Falsches zu machen. Das war richtig hart. @Das muss ich nie wieder haben@" (IP14: 330).

245 „[B]löderweise wirst Du auch nicht, äh sagen wir mal so, befördert zurück zu kommen. Man hat, im Gegenteil das Gefühl, dass man dort nicht mehr erwünscht ist. 'Da kommst Du jetzt aus Deutschland und was willst Du mir zeigen, he?' (…) Ne? So diese Art" (IP17: 336/338).

what we can and we talk to the patient very little, and I can't do that anymore (IP18: 407).[246]

Dr Elias Bähr, again, did not want to give up the financial position he acquired while working in Germany. Although his former head physician in the hospital he worked in prior to migration tried to win him back whenever Dr Bähr visited, so far he withstood this offer in spite of being tempted to work in his native language again. "I said, 'Ok, if I'll get the salary I received before, I won't come.' Every time, he offered a little more. Now we got up to 1000 Euro with shifts @(.)@" (IP28: 371).[247] Consequently, the migrant physicians were not ready to give up the ideals they had envisioned prior to, and achieved after migration, by returning to their home countries again.

At the same time, the respondents were not ready to stay under any circumstances. In spite of appreciating his financial situation in Germany, Dr Bähr, for instance, requested to be treated appropriately and stressed the importance of the recognition of his qualifications. When his skills were questioned by a nurse telling him that he was not entitled to do a night shift in the intensive care unit (see 5.2.6), he approached his head physician: "If you got a problem with me being new or a foreigner, no problem, I can leave" (IP28: 136).[248] Another aspect that encourages re-migration is the inclination to move closer to friends who also migrated to Germany (IP04: 197). Others might re-migrate after being recruited by head hunters, such as in the case of Dr Elena Eichhorn. "I also receive a lot of offers, also in [big city in Eastern Germany] and around" (IP09: 194).[249] Hence, after having achieved their primary goal of becoming a medical specialist, migrant physicians are likely to become more flexible themselves, and also attractive for other hospitals. They will then be familiar with the local professional and work culture, fluent in the German language, and trained specialists in their respective field.

In sum, the CEE migrant doctors' future plans were predominantly still very tentative and might never be implemented that way. Nevertheless, the expressed action orientations reveal that the migrant physicians perceived their stay in Germany primarily as a status passage to complete specialist training. Those who had established a family were more certain that they would remain in Germany rather than re-migrate. Singles that were determined to stay in Germany based this inclination on a potential loss of status and professional

---

246 „[J]etzt meine ganze Meinung [ist] anders. Also ich kann nicht mehr denken so einfach, weil in [meinem Heimatland] die Ärzte sind hier und die Patienten sind hier unten und äh ja, wir machen was wir können und wir reden mit dem Patient ganz wenig und das kann ich nicht mehr" (IP18: 407).

247 „Ich habe gesagt, 'OK wenn ich bekomme diese Gehalt was früher war, komme ich nicht.' Er sagt immer ein bisschen mehr. Jetzt wir sind bei 1000 Euro mit Di-, mit Dienst @(.)@" (IP28: 371).

248 „Wenn Sie haben damit Problem, dass ich neu bin oder Ausländer bin, kein Problem, ich kann weitergehen" (IP28: 136).

249 „[I]ch bekomme auch ganz viele Angebote auch in [Großstadt in Ostdeutschland] und in der Nähe" (IP09: 194).

ideals they have achieved by migrating to Germany and thus the fear of repeated uncertainty which they were eager to prevent. Hence, also for single migrant physicians the costs were too high. Nevertheless, this does not mean that all migrant physicians were eager to stay in the hospitals they are currently working in. Dissatisfaction on-site, as well as opportunities in professional or social terms that come up elsewhere (in Germany) might trigger them to leave. This high flexibility reflects the individualised post-accession migration patterns that were found to apply to CEE migrants in the UK (see ch. 3.1).

6.4 Interim conclusions

The goal of the present chapter was the depiction of the perspective of the CEE migrant physicians practicing in German hospitals. The findings are based on 21 problem-centred interviews with migrant physicians from Bulgaria, the Czech Republic, Hungary, Latvia, Poland, Romania and Slovakia. The analysis focused on how the migrant physicians perceived their migration to Germany, their employment in local hospitals, and how they coped with challenges and difficulties. The chapter was structured chronologically discussing the migrant physicians' *migration motivations and strategies*, initial *barriers and struggles* they encountered with respect to the transfer and application of their knowledge and skills, and finally their *balances and future plans* in reflection of the migration costs they had to face. The findings were discussed in the context of the results from the expert interviews presented in chapter 6. In this final subchapter I draw some interim conclusions with respect to the subordinate research questions.

CEE migrant physicians in German hospitals – a new form of East-West migration?

Corresponding to the concept of 'normal life' (Galasińska & Kozłowska, 2009), the main motivation of the CEE migrant physicians under study to migrate to Germany was the envisioned possibility of a 'normal career' as medical doctor. Normality in this respect referred to the institutional and ethical conception of the medical profession and a physician's role. This included both health care provision and medical practice according to the medical ethos and the latest medical standards, as well as the expectation of a stable job and financial security. Like in post-accession migration to the UK, also the migrant doctors in the sample migrated mainly for work. However, in the typology of Trevena (2013), they would fall into the category of "career seekers", since the migrant doctors had the concrete aim to earn better, to gain work experience, and to advance in their own profession. More diffuse migration motives in terms of the general aim to earn more, or to gain work experience abroad, irrespective of the actual occupational field, which Trevena (ibid.) described as typical for "drifters" and "target earners" were not stated in the case under study. Nevertheless, one has to bear in mind, that the sample only consisted of migrant physicians working in hospitals, and thus excluded CEE physicians who potentially migrated to Germany as "drifters" or "target earners" making money in other jobs or as fee-based physicians.

As Engbersen and Snel (2013) found the medical migration from CEE to Germany is not based on a migration scheme, but undertaken individually. Nonetheless, it is strongly demand-driven, as expressed by the HR managers and medical directors above (ch. 5.1). This is also reflected in the migrant doctors' migration strategies. Hence, both the institutionalised infrastructure of recruitment agencies and job fairs, as well as the professional networks of CEE migrant physicians already working in Germany directly resulted from the shortage of physicians in German hospitals. These conditions facilitated migration and reduced migration costs.

Another consequence of the demand of physicians, and at the same time the most crucial aspect in which this medical migration to Germany seems to differ from post-accession East-West migration to the UK, is the fact that these migrant doctors are placed at the primary labour market. They work under the same structural conditions as their German (-trained) colleagues, as the HR managers, medical directors and migrant physicians confirmed in the interviews. Nevertheless, as stated in previous research (Kovacheva & Grewe, 2015b) and by the interviewed HR managers and medical directors (ch. 5.1), the demand for migrant physicians is highest in rural areas, whereas city hospitals by and large still manage to recruit German (-trained) physicians. Accordingly, although some of the migrant physicians under study stated to have intentionally chosen a small facility, it is obvious that these migrant physicians fill those positions that German (-trained) physicians reject. Hence, as observed in the UK and diagnosed for CEE migrants in Western European countries in general (Favell, 2008b), also in this case, the CEE migrants do the jobs that natives do not accept.

Although statements about the length of the migrant doctors' stay cannot be made with certainty, the interviewees' accounts imply that this medical migration to Germany tends to be more long term than previous post-accession migration from CEE to the UK. This might be due to the fact that "career seekers" (Trevena, 2013) are more established at the local labour market, and thus more inclined to stay. Nevertheless, some of the migrant doctors were still unsure about whether to remain in Germany beyond residency. They perceived their stay in Germany primarily as a status passage, a necessary step to take in order to proceed in their professional career. They will make the final decision about their subsequent plans later on. Thus, as outlined by Parutis (2014), their initial aspiration of completing residency in Germany and then potentially moving on could transform into the wish to settle down in Germany. Irrespective of the final outcome and tendency, the common ground that the post-accession migration to the UK and this medical migration to Germany have, is the migrants' ability to be flexible in this respect which is primarily due to the CEE migrants status as 'EU movers'.

Hence, while some aspects of the migration of CEE physicians to Germany reflect the patterns of post-accession of East-West migration to the UK, others are diametrically different. In any case, the migration trend under study gives visibility to CEE migrants as highly skilled EU movers, and thus adds to the diversity of forms of mobility.

The migrant physicians' perception of and way of coping with their situation in the German hospitals

Despite the uncomplicated legality for CEE migrant physicians to practice in Germany, they encountered a number of different barriers that impaired the transfer of their professional knowledge and skills. Consequently, their professional self-concept and status in the new work environment suffered. Altogether, five main obstacles were identified.

First, although the formal recognition of university credentials to obtain the medical license was uncomplicated in most cases, the formal recognition of previously completed years of specialist training abroad, posed difficulties to the migrant doctors. These difficulties did not only consist of the reluctance of the responsible medical association to recognise these qualifications as equal, but in the lack of information provided about the recognition procedure on the part of the hospital administration. In these cases, migrant doctors were employed under their qualifications, which only one respondent vehemently complained about.

Second, different forms of tacit knowledge impeded the direct transfer of the migrant doctors' professional knowledge and skills. Tacit knowledge encompasses, on the one hand, "encultured knowledge" (Collins, 1993) with regard to the situational language competence (Bourdieu, 2009). In spite of having past the required German test, the migrant physicians initially had difficulties in communicating in German. On the other hand, tacit knowledge pertained to the local work and professional culture. Having been professionally and culturally socialised abroad, they were not familiar with local codes of conduct and ways of approaching certain tasks and examinations. As a consequence, the migrant physicians were not able to directly apply their expertise and know-how, and thus to fulfil their role as medical doctor.

Third, their inability to fulfil the role as physician threatened their professional identity. Due to the unfamiliarity with the local customs and procedures, the migrant doctors were not able to perform all tasks independently and take over full responsibilities for their patients. Consequently, they failed to transfer their professional self-concept. This dissatisfaction with the own performance was partially based on social norms of the medical profession that pose certain expectations towards the role of a physician. Based on the high identification of physicians with their profession, not fulfilling these norms, such as clinical autonomy (Allsop & Mulcahy, 1998), as well as omnipotence and omniscience (Helmreich & Merritt, 2008), and the requirement of a competent appearance (Pfadenhauer, 2003), caused them major indisposition. This posed a threat to their professional identity (cp. Bernstein, 2000), and at the same time questioned the purpose of their migration which was in most cases strongly oriented towards advancement in the medical career. Consequently, these difficulties put the migrant doctors in existential struggles.

Fourth, this uncertainty was fuelled by social expectations on the part of colleagues and superiors based on the circumstances of pressing staff shortages. Since the migrant doctors were recruited in order to meet the demand, they were expected to take work off their hands immediately, and without extensive incorporation measures, as stated by the HR managers and medical directors (ch. 5.4.3). Hence, the responsibility to become familiar with the new work environment was predominantly transferred to the individual migrant physician, who was confronted with high expectations to quickly fill the gap, proceed according to the local work culture, and take work off their colleagues' hands. In this respect, the expressed preference of HR managers and medical directors for migrant physicians who resemble German (-trained) physicians to the largest degree possible, helps to understand the pressure, the migrant physicians felt exposed to. Being overstrained with the situation, the lack of support on the part of the hospital administration and other staff added to the uncertainty caused by the unfamiliar workplace and the difficulties applying their skills. The example of the few physicians who enjoyed an intensive incorporation, and gained confidence from this induction feeling ready to take over full responsibilities earlier than others, supports this claim.

Fifth, the devaluation of the migrant physicians' professional qualifications based on mistrust and disrespect contributed to their uncertainty. This was shown to them particularly by nurses, and in a few cases, also colleagues, superiors, and patients. Their social expectations towards the physicians were perceived by the respondents to be based on attributes such as experience, age, nationality, and the fact that they did not complete their studies in Germany. Supporting the finding of Bernstein (2000) that not only the own certainty that they can master their responsibilities is crucial for physicians' professional self-esteem, but also approval on the part of others, the interviewees suffered from the perceived lack of recognition.

Taken together, these barriers resulted in a perceived loss of status as medical doctor on the part of the migrant physicians both based dissatisfaction with their own performance, as well as lack of recognition and out-spoken praise by others. It confronted the migrant doctors with a sense of failure on the one hand because it questioned their capability as physicians and on the other because it questioned their migration, which was meant to serve the purpose of career advancement. In order to compensate for this uncertainty, the migrant physicians applied different forms of "biographical certainty strategies" (Zinn, 2004). In terms of *certainty constructions* (ibid.) they distanced themselves from the nurses by applying an interpretation of the situation according to the inter-professional order they were used to from their countries of origin, and they rationalised incidences of discrimination in order to overshadow unpleasant situations which they perceived as threat to both their professional self-concept and their migration decision. With regard to *protective action* (ibid.), migrant physicians were eager to adjust themselves as soon as possible to the local work environment and professional order by own means, and stated action orientations for the future that would prevent a repeated situation of uncertainty.

First of all, the migrant doctors encountered tensions with the nurses who did not respect the superior status of the migrant physicians in the professional hierarchy and refused to follow the physicians' instructions or interfered with their decisions based on their experiences. The migrant physicians perceived this as undermining their authority and as devaluation of their competence. In order to counter this affront, some of the physicians reinterpreted the situation by stressing their expertise vis-á-vis the nurses' practical knowledge, and by applying professional standards from the medical systems they were trained in, in which nurses have broader responsibilities. Hence, they degraded the local nurses' tasks and thereby mentally constructed certainty based on their regained superior status.

Moreover, the migrant physicians employed the certainty strategy of rationalisation, another *certainty construction* (Zinn, 2004), in which the migrant physicians re-interpreted unfavourable situations, for instance, in which they experienced symbolic exclusion, by adapting their expectations so that no notion of failure occurred. Rationalising such situations by declaring them as normal and expected – at least for the initial phase, or degrading the nurses' tasks to highlight the own position, the physicians covered up their disappointment or dissatisfaction with the situation. Referring to this exclusion as bound to a particular temporary phase, or pointing to the limitations of the nurses' responsibilities, they diverted the attention from their perceived lack of recognition. Thus, they annulled the questioning of their migration and legitimised it by constructing an assessable and thus certain scenario.

Another coping strategy that the migrant doctors employed was the one of adjustment aimed at quickly establishing the lacking certainty through *protective action* (Zinn, 2004). Realising that they could not smoothly transfer their professional skills and knowledge to the new working environment, the migrant physicians made an effort to quickly learn and adapt to the local work culture in order to re-establish their status as physician. Since autonomy is a crucial part of a physicians' professional identity (Allsop & Mulcahy, 1998), and the expectation of colleagues that physicians will "pull their own weight," they did not want to ask for help. Rather, they wanted to prove their capability to themselves and others. Therefore, they worked long hours or secretly took paper work home, in order to not be a burden to others and thus reveal their dependence and inability to complete tasks in time. That way, the migrant doctors re-established their status towards others, and reassured their professional identity for their own self-esteem.

Finally, the migrant doctors expressed their action orientation to remain in Germany, another strategy of *protective action* (Zinn, 2004). Once having managed to obtain recognition in their capacity as physician in Germany, they were not ready to give this up again by re-migrating to their home or another country. Instead, they were eager to maintain their achievement as the result of a major status investment by staying in Germany. Re-migration would incur costs related to a de-valuing of their acquired skills in Germany, and more importantly, the issue of having to gain familiarity and language proficiency in a new cultural context; they would have to start anew getting used to a new working environment and a new language. On the other hand, this applied to the potential loss of aspects the migrant doctors appreciated, and that had initially motivated their migration, such as the medical standards in German hospitals or the financial stability they gained on-site. In that case, they perceived that their migration and the related struggle would have been to no purpose. In this respect, the migrant doctors drew on their "transnational orientation as biographical resource" (Nowicka, 2014) informing their orientation to remain in Germany based on their embedding in two different social contexts, the one of the former and the current country of residence. Therefore, their action orientations with respect to their future life choices was on norms of, and expectations towards a 'normal life' (Galasińska & Kozłowska, 2009) from different places, enabling the migrant doctors to assess the option of staying in Germany as more favourable than the one of return migration. In both cases, the one of re-migration to another country, and the one of return migration, they would again be confronted with a phase of uncertainty.

A final factor of this strategy is the one of the physicians' stage in the life course. Those with a family extended the notion of *protective action* (Zinn, 2004) from themselves to their spouse and children. They argued that they wanted to stay in Germany in order not to put their spouse and children in a situation again, in which they would have to struggle with uncertainty in terms of a new language and a new environment. Singles, however, stated that their decision on where to live and work in the future would depend on where they find a partner. On the one hand, this shift in priorities with regard to the motive of future migration compared to the one for this initial migration from professional to private life, can be explained with the common order of life stages (e.g. Vysotskaya, 2011). On the other hand, from the perspective of *protective action* (Zinn, 2004), this choice can be interpreted as yet another strategy to avoid uncertainty, however, not with regard to experienced indisposition in terms of professional difficulties, but in terms of social migration costs.

In sum, the CEE migrant physicians experienced a number of barriers upon arrival in the German hospitals that particularly during their initial phase on-site led to major uncertainties based on implications from their professional ethos, and social expectations based on the pressing staff situation in the hospitals. The physicians addressed these challenges with the help of different strategies aimed at restoring certainty. Those who had overcome this phase at the time of the interview perceived these efforts as an investment to advance their professional status, and tended to be against re-migration. Additionally, those who were still in the middle of this professional and private acculturation struggle, still evaluated their migration as worthwhile given the situation in their former countries of residence, and were preponderantly oriented towards remaining in Germany.

"Ensuring access and promotion is both: a question of justice and a gain for society"
(Federal President Joachim Gauck, 2014) [250]

7 Conclusions

In this dissertation I researched the migration of CEE physicians to Germany and their recruitment to and incorporation in German hospitals highlighting institutional strategies on the part of hospital administrations on the one hand, and the experience thereof by the migrant physicians on the other. By focussing on a group of migrants enjoying extensive mobility rights due to their status as EU citizens and highly-skilled, my primary empirical contribution is determining and highlighting the insufficiency of policy level changes alone in ensuring a satisfied and sustainable highly skilled migrant work force. My research results emphasise that factors such as hands-on training and informal recognition are playing a pivotal role in the workplace integration of migrant physicians. These factors are severely impacting personal employment satisfaction, productivity, and a willingness to commit to a long-term integration into German society. While currently tolerated due to unfavourable circumstances in other countries, policy changes in those countries may easily render Germany considerably less competitive in the labour market of highly-skilled physicians, which is beyond Germany's control. More importantly, irrespective of labour shortages, highly competent migrants are not being given an appropriate platform to exercise and further develop their skills, and are being significantly underutilised and unsupported in key aspects, which is an inherently undesirable situation from the perspective of both the migrant physicians themselves and the German medical profession.

The stance of the German government towards immigration in general, and immigration of CEE migrants in particular, has undergone a drastic change. Germany has developed from being traditionally restrictive to being one of the most liberal countries in terms of immigration policies for highly skilled migrants (OECD, 2013). Against this backdrop, I was interested in how far this opening on the policy level reflected in the recruitment and incorporation of the migrant physicians in the hospital routine. In order to answer this general research question, I subdivided it into two subordinate questions asking for the nature of this new form of East-West migration to Germany, as well

---

250 „Einstieg und Aufstieg zu gewährleisten, ist beides: eine Frage der Gerechtigkeit und ein Gewinn für die Gesellschaft" (Federal President Joachim Gauck, Speech from May 22, 2014, naturalisation celebration on the occasion of the 65th anniversary of the German Basic Law. Own translation.).

as the perception thereof on the part of the CEE migrant physicians. To this end, I chose a qualitative exploratory approach. With respect to the first subordinate research question, I included two different perspectives. Firstly, I accounted for the perspective of the hospital administrations in order to gain knowledge about the process of the recruitment and induction, as well as collectively shared interpretation patterns concerning the situation. Secondly, I accounted for the perspective of the CEE migrant physicians, focussing on their migration motives and strategies. With regard to the second subordinate research question, I applied the conceptual approach of "biographical uncertainty" (Zinn, 2010). I collected the data by conducting nine expert interviews with HR managers and medical directors from seven different hospitals in German urban and rural areas, and 21 problem-centred interviews with male and female migrant physicians from the Czech Republic, Bulgaria, Hungary, Latvia, Poland, Romania, and Slovakia working in the same hospitals as the HR managers and medical directors. The expert interviews were analysed using deductive and inductive codes, the problem-centred interviews were analysed with the help of different coding techniques with regard to the descriptive findings. In order to analyse interpretative patterns and coping strategies, the three step coding technique used in Grounded Theory was applied.

In this concluding chapter, I briefly summarise the main findings of the two empirical chapters (ch. 5 and 6) in light of the two subsequent research questions before discussing them against the backdrop of the general research question that has been guiding my study. I continue with the consideration of critical issues and suggestions for future research, and end with some final reflections.

The nature of the migration of CEE physicians to Germany

The first subordinate research question focussed on the circumstances of the migration of CEE medical doctors to Germany. Its first dimension was targeted at how the recruitment and induction of the migrant physicians are organised on the part of the hospital administrations. The findings revealed differences between the seven hospitals included in the sample with regard to demand and recruitment strategies representing their size and location, as well as tensions with regard to the HR managers' and medical directors' attitude towards the recruitment of physicians from abroad. First of all, while HR managers and medical directors of the city hospitals stated to only occasionally rely on migrant physicians, those of rural hospitals declared that without migrant physicians they could not keep the hospital running. Accordingly, HR managers and medical directors of city hospitals did not actively engage in recruitment from abroad, but were able to meet their demand with traditional recruitment strategies. HR managers and medical directors of rural hospitals, however, became active in recruiting from abroad and were more systematic in their recruitment strategies. Additionally, with regard to incorporation measures, rural hospitals were better attuned to welcoming migrant physicians on-site in terms of accommodation, assistance with bureaucracy, and the provision of language classes.

Nevertheless, HR managers and medical directors of both urban and rural hospitals were by and large dissatisfied with their facilities' dependency on migrant physicians. They wished for an internal solution initiated by the German government, and did not regard the liberalisation of access regulations to the medical license for migrant physicians as a legitimate way to address the shortage. Nevertheless, HR managers and medical directors recruited migrant physicians out of necessity. Only a few of the respondents had accepted the situation and regarded the incorporation of the migrant doctors as being of mutual interest. The majority, however, had very high expectations towards the CEE migrant doctors. They expected them to function immediately in order to fill the vacancy, but an intensive induction into the local work routine to ensure a quick adjustment was rarely provided. Thus, the fact that these physicians were socialised in different medical systems was neglected. Therefore, the HR managers' and medical directors' recruitment and induction practices did not appear sustainable.

The second dimension of the first subordinate research question dealt with how the migrant physicians conceive their migration in terms of motivations and expectations, and which migration strategies they apply. It shows that their major intention was normality of their professional life regarding training and working conditions, but also institutional and ethical conceptions of the medical profession in terms of medical practice and the provision of medical care. They oriented these visions towards both the latest medical standards and the medical ethos. The migrant physicians perceived the shortage in Germany as a window of opportunity to realise their professional ideals, without which the majority would not have embarked on emigration. The institutional infrastructure for recruitment as well as the already existing professional networks of CEE physicians in Germany facilitated the migration and enabled their positioning at the primary labour market. Although some of the migrant physicians were still undecided about the length of their stay, most of them indicated their wish to stay in Germany as a long-term strategy.

Overall, the migration of CEE physicians to Germany is clearly demand-driven. The demand for migrant physicians on the part of German hospitals reflects in the CEE migrant doctors' motives to choose Germany as a destination country as well as in their migration strategies, relying on infrastructure that has developed due to the shortage of physicians. Consequently, these CEE migrants did not migrate with the diffuse aims of somehow earning money, or improving language skills and gaining international experience while working abroad. Instead, they had the concrete goal to advance in their careers as physicians. Additionally, the fact that they are employed as physicians and being positioned at the primary labour market in such large numbers results from the pressing shortage and the dependence of the German hospital administrations on the migrant doctors.

Despite these conditions, this medical migration shares common features with both post-accession East-West migration to the UK, as well as with previous East-West migration to Germany. These features are, first of all, the individuality of migration strategies, irrespective of the demand-driven character, as well as the flexibility of the migrants reflected in their open future plans. This is mainly due to the migrants' status as intra-EU movers, which enables them to make short-term decisions and to base these on their experiences abroad, as well as personal factors that might become crucial at a later point in time. These circumstances put CEE migrants in a more powerful position than they used to be in. However, another common feature is that, as with other CEE migrants in Germany and other parts of Western Europe, they are employed in jobs that natives reject. This applies to the CEE migrant doctors in German hospitals in terms of the location of their jobs. As Kovacheva and Grewe (2015b) found for the case of Hamburg, city hospitals prefer, and are still able to rely on, German (-trained) physicians, or at least those migrant physicians who previously gained work experience in a German hospital. This matches my finding that rural hospitals in particular have to actively recruit from abroad. Correspondingly, CEE migrant physicians are predominantly employed in remote, rural areas that German (-trained) physicians find unattractive.

The CEE migrant physicians' perception of their situation in German hospitals

The CEE migrant doctors were mostly satisfied with the uncomplicated bureaucratic procedures, the structural conditions and medical standards they met in the German hospitals. Many of them, additionally, spoke positively about their relationships to colleagues, superiors, and patients. However, despite the favourable starting conditions, they encountered a number of barriers and challenges upon arrival in the German hospitals, which they perceived as a devaluation of their cultural capital and loss of status as medical doctor. First, while the formal recognition of credentials was uncomplicated, at least for those who had recently arrived in Germany, the formal recognition of previously completed years of residency was not readily granted. Furthermore, the hospital administrations had been very supportive with regard to bureaucratic procedures required to obtain the medical license. Thus, the physicians fulfilled the prerequisite to practice medicine, and the hospital administration could fill their vacancy. However, they were less helpful with regard to the recognition of completed years of specialist training. Second, different forms of tacit knowledge impeded the direct transfer of professional knowledge and skills.

This applied both to the local work culture and professional order as well as to situational components of language proficiency in terms of social customs of interaction. Third, due to this limitation, the migrant doctors had trouble in fulfilling their envisioned role of a physician since they were not able to perform their tasks independently and were afraid not to appear competently in their profession. This limited their self-esteem and created discomfort. Fourth, most of the CEE migrant physicians lacked support on the part of the hospital administration or colleagues that would have helped them to faster become familiar with the local work culture. Fifth, some of the physicians experienced incidences of symbolic exclusion on the part of colleagues, nurses, and patients. They refused to cooperate with them, or be treated by them, respectively, based on mistrust in their competence as physicians. This mistrust was partly triggered by the migrant doctors' deficiencies in the German language, but also by stereotypes. Taken together, these devaluations complicated the migrant physicians' transfer of their professional knowledge and skills to the German hospitals, and left them with the notion of failure in both their capacity as medical doctors, as well as the purpose of their migration.

In order to compensate for these devaluations, and to re-establish certainty, the migrant physicians applied different strategies. First, they applied "certainty constructions" (Zinn, 2004) by degrading nurses and re-interpreting expectations through rationalising perceived devaluations. Thereby, they constructed a match between their expectations and their experiences on-site, hence, re-establishing biographical certainty. Second, they employed "protective action" (ibid.). They coped with the impediments of their performance based on unfamiliarity with the local work culture and communication habits by making an effort to quickly and independently adjust to local standards and requirements. In this way they proved their capability and re-gained trust in their professional abilities both on the part of others as well as of themselves. Additionally, they were eager to avoid situations of uncertainty in the future by stating the action orientation to stay in Germany in order to not lose the hard-won informal recognition through return or re-migration to countries, in which different standards and requirements apply, and their status investment would again be devalued. Only one migrant physician considered re-migrating to his home country or another country due to a perceived lack of informal recognition.

The CEE migrant doctors' action orientation with regard to future plans was additionally informed by both a "double frame of reference" (Nowicka, 2012) towards home and host country, as well as by the migrant doctors' stages in their life course. With regard to the former, the migrant physicians drew on their "transnational orientation as biographical resource" (Nowicka, 2014). Knowing about the primarily professional conditions in both their previous and current country of residence, they based their evaluations of their situation in the German hospitals on a vision of *normality* that was informed by norms from at least two national contexts. Hence, in spite of experienced devaluations, they assessed their situation on-site as better than in their home countries. Furthermore, their stage in the life course impacted their decision in terms of prioritising private over professional plans after having finished residency, and of considering not only their own needs, but also the needs and migration costs of other family members in making future migration decisions.

The migration of CEE migrant physicians to Germany in the light of liberalised immigration policies and access regulations to the medical profession

The general research question addressed potentially remaining limitations to the mobility of migrant physicians in German hospitals. The liberalisation of immigration policies and access barriers for migrant physicians in practicing medicine vis-á-vis the shortage of physicians in Germany showed a positive effect. This outcome finds its expression in the massive facilitations in terms of bureaucratic procedures, the numbers of CEE migrant doctors coming to Germany, the fact that most of them state to be overall satisfied with their migration decision, and plan to remain in Germany. Hence, superficially, the medical migration of CEE migrant physicians to Germany appears to be a both-win situation. However, further investigation reveals that the qualities of the motives of the German hospital administrations to recruit migrant physicians on the one hand, and most of the CEE doctors' motivations to migrate to Germany on the other, are diametrically opposed. While the former wish to maintain the functionality of their facilities and depend on a smooth transfer of knowledge and skills on the part of the recruited doctors, the latter hope to receive an encompassing specialist training. Accordingly, the CEE migrant physicians encountered a number of adversities and barriers that went beyond the formal recognition of their credentials and the reception of the medical license. Consequently, the liberalisation of policies and access regulations proved to be a necessary, but not sufficient measure to sustainably attract and incorporate migrant doctors. This finding is outlined in the following aspects.

First, there has been a tremendous development with regard to the formal recognition of foreign medical credentials. Restricted issuance of the German medical license has been liberalized in response to the increasing shortage of physicians in Germany. However, although the EU directive 36/2005/EC on the recognition of professional qualifications is supposed to ensure the smooth transfer of professional qualifications, barriers remain with regard to formal, as well as informal recognition thereof. Difficulties occur, for instance, with regard to the recognition of previously completed years of specialist training. The defined expertise a physician of a certain medical field is expected to master, again, depends on the country where the training took place, and even varied between the different Laender within Germany. Hence, irrespective of the freedom of movement and the harmonisation directive, critical barriers remain within the medical profession expressing its reluctance to open up for migrant doctors. These institutional barriers are constructed on the part of the medical association striving to retain the prerequisite of interpretation and their power as a self-governed institution despite losses in light of the growing demand (see ch. 2.2.3). The question remains whether this closure would change with an increased demand of advanced junior physicians and medical specialists in German hospitals, urging for a faster processing time. However, again this would likely be an enforced rather than a deliberate opening.

Second, an aspect that cannot be catered for by the liberalisation of immigration policies and access regulations to the medical profession is the attitude of the hospital administrations recruiting migrant physicians. Being confronted with the recruitment of physicians from abroad as the sole solution to address the pressing staff situation in their facilities, they see themselves trapped between the need of keeping the day-to-day-business running, and the impossibility of the migrant physicians' frictionless transfer to the German work environment. Therefore, the HR managers and medical directors make an effort to recruit migrant physicians and to help them take up employment quickly in order to fill the facility's vacancy. However, they are reluctant in supporting the migrant physicians in becoming familiar with the local work routine in an extensive way that would require them to initially cut down their working hours since this would not meet the demand. The sentiment that therefore the recruitment of doctors from abroad is not an adequate solution finds expression in the requirement of German language proficiency, which the respondents highlighted most with regard to recruitment criteria. The necessity that migrant physicians are fluent in German is tirelessly stressed, while at the same time HR managers and medical directors admit that oftentimes the staff situation is so pressing that they are not in the position to be overly selective. Together with the experience of the migrant physicians that they learn the language best by being exposed to its usage in the daily hospital routine, this language issue, which appears as a logical and understandable argument, can thus be understood as a constructed barrier that serves as a pretext to prove the perceived inadequacy to address the shortage in this way. The hospital administrations expose the problems of the lacking proficiency in German, but are reluctant to actually tackle the issue in an adequate way.

As a consequence of this reluctant attitude, the HR managers and medical directors, who are primarily concerned with the hospitals' interests, tend to neglect the needs of the migrant physicians and confront them with high expectations. Other than in the case of the guest workers (see ch. 2.1.1), measures are taken to assist the migrant physicians in getting settled on-site and also making the accompanying family feel at home. Nonetheless, like linguistic incorporation, also an intensive professional induction helping them to quickly find their way in the local work routine is missing in most cases. The HR managers and medical directors – whether for economic or ideological reasons – neglect the fact that the migrant physicians were socialised in different medical systems, and that the differing work and professional cultures pose initial barriers to the physicians' transfer of professional knowledge and skills. The incorporation of the migrant physicians is thus conceived as a one-way-street in which the main burden of integration is assigned to the migrant physicians. Consequently, in some cases, these functional priorities fall short in providing the physicians with the encompassing specialist training for which they migrated to Germany. These circumstances bear the risk of wearing out and exploiting the migrant physicians, and reveal a lack of intensive engagement with their sustainable recruitment.

Third, despite the liberalisation of policies and regulations, the transfer of tacit knowledge such as codes of conduct and standard approaches to medical procedures remains problematic. Since these are not considered in the harmonisation of professional qualifications (see also Jefferies & Evetts, 2000), they differ between hospitals and medical systems. These differences complicate the initial phase of the migrant physicians in the German hospitals with regard to the cooperation with colleagues and nurses, as well as the interaction with patients. Due to their institutionalised character, expectations of the migrant physicians' performance on the part of the named groups were shaped by local professional standards and norms. Accordingly, migrant physicians felt that they were denied informal recognition in their capacities as medical doctors on the part of colleagues, nurses, and patients, unless they adhered to these precise approaches. Hence, failing in the "competence to represent competence" (Pfadenhauer, 2003), their qualifications were devalued in acts of symbolic exclusion. These were based on mistrust towards their knowledge and skills, national stereotypes, and with respect to colleagues and nurses, the fear of additional work in times of an already pressing staff situation. Instead of providing the migrant doctors with an intensive induction in their initial phase onsite, which would accelerate and shorten the period in which their support was required, some of them made the incorporation additionally hard for them. Hence, barriers were again constructed that reveal prejudice and a lack of openness towards migrant physicians also on this individual level.

Taken together, all three shortcomings with regard to the incorporation of the migrant physicians that exist in spite of the liberalised immigration policies and access regulations to the medical profession highlight the relative nature of professional qualifications. The barriers were constructed and held up based on the endeavour to retain power, on economic considerations, or on the fear of additional work. In any case, they imply a continuance of a previously known reluctance towards immigrants on the part of German society. This attitude is emphasised by the understanding of incorporation as a one-way-street, and the corresponding lack of sufficient incorporation measures in most of the hospitals.

In the case of the CEE migrant physicians this strategy works out. Despite experiencing major barriers and the perceived devaluation in their status as medical doctors, the majority of the CEE migrant physicians under study expressed satisfaction with their migration decision, as well as the working and training conditions in the German hospitals. This evaluation was strongly driven by the knowledge of the respective conditions in their home countries and former countries of residence, as well as vis-á-vis the restricted opportunities to complete specialist training in other Western countries. Consequently, instead of complaining about their situation, the CEE migrant doctors made an effort to quickly adapt to local standards without demanding help or assistance. Therefore, the German hospital administrations benefited from the migrant physicians' wish for career advancement under envisioned professional conditions, and the lack of possibilities to find these conditions elsewhere. Nevertheless, HR managers and medical directors are ill advised to rely on these circumstances. As soon as conditions in the physicians' home countries improve, or access to specialist training in countries such as the UK gets liberalised, German hospitals are likely to lose attractiveness for the CEE migrant physicians. Due to their EU citizenship, they have the independence and flexibility to migrate elsewhere within the EU. Hospital administrations would have to make a considerably more concerted effort if they intended to ensure a sustainable recruitment and incorporation of migrant physicians, being exposed to the international "race for the best minds" (Nohl & Weiß, 2011).

Critical issues and suggestions for future research

Drawing these conclusions, there are a few caveats that require consideration and provide implications for future research. Firstly, I conducted interviews only with those CEE migrant physicians who were employed in a German hospital at the time of the interviews. Consequently, it can be assumed that these physicians were by and large satisfied with their situation. In order to gain a deeper or more encompassing insight into which factors drive return or re-migration, it would be useful to include physicians who left before or after having completed specialist training in a German hospital. Although three physicians in my sample had worked in other German hospitals before, I did not focus on the reasons for why they had left the previous facility they had worked in.

Secondly, ex-post questions on initial migration motives and expectations are always problematic. Experiences in the host country might have changed or distorted initial motivations and considerations. In a similar vein this applies to questions about future plans. Experiences the migrants have later on might alter initial plans so that those expressed might not come true. Therefore, a longitudinal study with at least three times of inquiry – one prior to, one after migration, and another one, for instance, after having completed residency – would help to get a more concise view on the entire migration and integration process.

Another suggestion for future research is to include migrant physicians from Western EU member countries. Focusing on CEE migrant doctors, I gathered detailed information on the circumstances of their migration and their experiences in Germany. However, in order to be able to provide a systematic evaluation of their situation, and of the assumption that CEE highly skilled migrants are a special group based on previous patterns of East-West migration to Germany and Europe in general, a comparison with other groups of migrant doctors would be useful. Since Kovacheva and Grewe (2015b) whose sample consisted mainly of non-EU physicians had similar findings with regard to the difficulties of incorporation at the work place, it would be instructive to draw comparisons with the situation of migrant physicians of an assumedly higher social prestige in Germany, such as migrants from Western EU member countries (Gerhards & Lengfeld, 2009).

Furthermore, the findings revealed that membership in the medical profession and the identification with the role of a medical doctor was a crucial component in the migrant physicians' motivation to migrate, as well as the evaluation of their experiences on-site. Therefore, a comparison with migrants in other professional and occupational fields would help to assess to what extent implications can be transferred to the incorporation of skilled and highly skilled migrants in other professions and occupations.

Some of the aspects that I was interested in did not prove to be fruitful during the interviews. This pertained to the question of gender differences, or the organisation of migrant physicians in the respective unions. As reasons, I identified the early stage of their career, the recent arrival, and, relatedly, their occupation with more acute problems of finding their way during this initial phase (see ch. 4.5). Research focusing on these aspects with regard to migrant physicians at a later stage of their employment in German hospitals taking up these topics might be more yielding. The findings would contribute to research on the current topic of the feminisation of medicine (Heru, 2005) from an intersectional perspective, and to strengthening the position of migrant physicians in German hospitals in general.

Since the data on migrant physicians in Germany is very poor (see ch. 2.2.3), it is impossible to assess, for instance, at which stage of their career migrant physicians tend to arrive in Germany, how long they stay, whether they tend to specialise in specific fields and so on. Improved quantitative data would help to better understand and monitor their migration, and to develop adequate measures to ensure their incorporation.

Wider implications for the medical profession and Germany as a country of immigration

The findings show that openness towards foreign qualifications and professional standards particularly support familiarisation with local codes of conduct and cultural modes, including a situational language competence. Informal recognition and the appreciation of migrants' knowledge and skills are crucial for their incorporation at the workplace. On a structural level, openness towards foreign qualifications is expressed in the formal recognition of the migrant doctors' credentials and uncomplicated bureaucratic procedures. Nonetheless, the circumstances are not ideal, but there are measures that could improve the situation. First of all, medical standards and codes of conduct are still strongly nationally shaped leading to barriers for the immediate transfer of professional knowledge and skills across borders. In Germany, certain medical standards vary additionally between the different Laender, which is reflected in the differing curricula of medical studies. However, in 2014 both representatives of the German Medical Students Association and the German Council of Science and Humanities ("Wissenschaftsrat") declared themselves in favour of the standardisation of medical curricula throughout Germany (bvmd, 2014; Wissenschaftsrat, 2014). This would be a first step towards a more open profession that migrant physicians could also benefit from. With uniform standards mobility within Germany would increase. This increase in mobility would force medical associations to become acclimated with variations in professional conduct and more tolerant to physicians who are working in a medical system they have not been socialised in. This would clearly benefit migrants who naturally exhibit differing socialised norms.

Another recommendation for the further development of medical studies in Germany, that was stated by the Council of Science and Humanities, is the integration of course units on psychosocial and communicative skills and an earlier enabling of patient contact during the physicians' training. Through this measure, the practical orientation of medical training would be strengthened (ibid.). Migrant physicians who completed their studies abroad will not be able to benefit from this practical training directly. Nevertheless, again, the recollection of these interaction skills could increase the awareness for the fact that migrant physicians, in particular, who have been socialised in a different professional culture and in a different medical system require more experience in such communication and interaction skills. Making an effort to familiarise migrant physicians with these tacit aspects of medical knowledge and supporting them therein would improve the situation for all parties involved.

Apart from these aspects specified for the medical profession, my findings have implications that go beyond medicine. They are crucial with regard to the recruitment and incorporation of other skilled and highly skilled migrants to meet the demand in other occupational fields such as engineering, information technology or in trade. In all of these occupations, an open and supportive climate is required to incorporate migrants. This also applies to the informal recognition of migrants' knowledge and skills. The case of the migrant physicians showed how crucial the appreciation of their capabilities in their profession by others was to their professional identity and self-esteem. This finding links to the topic of an intercultural opening of fields such as public administration in which – despite the high number of migrants living in Germany – only very few migrants and their descendants are represented. An immigration country such as Germany hosting a diverse society and being dependent on further immigration, cannot afford to ignore the benefit and enrichment it could gain from these unexploited potentials.

In the same vein, this applies to the ban on employment for asylum seekers in Germany. Currently, large shares of refugees coming to Germany are skilled and highly skilled in occupations and professions that Germany is looking for. However, they are not allowed to take up employment while not having obtained a residence permit. Consequently, their potentials are not being used for months, and the asylum seekers feel useless for not being able to work, be independent and contribute to, as well as participate in society. A sign of recognition would be a programme of assessing their qualifications and preparing them for the German labour market, as is currently done in a pilot project run by the Federal Employment Agency and the Federal Office for Migration and Refugees in six German cities. Appreciating migrants' knowledge and skills, and valuing their additional language skills and their tacit knowledge in the form of their own migration experience, does not only make them feel welcome and valuable in society; their participation in the labour market would increase their acceptance in German society and thus contribute not only to the reduction of the sense of social exclusion on the part of migrants, but also to the reduction of prejudices on the part of German society.

Hence, by creating an open and supportive climate, and appreciating immigrants' knowledge and skills, Germany could complete its considerable development from not admitting its de-facto status as a country of immigration to being an immigration country with the promoted culture of welcoming immigrants and appreciating their abilities ("Willkommens- und Anerkennungskultur").

Final reflections

In this work, I "tested" the limits of the mobility of highly skilled migrants against the backdrop of liberalised immigration policies and access regulations to the German labour market. One the one hand, I chose the medical profession, which is traditionally self-contained, restrictive towards migrant physicians and yet suffers staff shortages; on the other hand I chose a group of migrants that, particularly in the German context, unites contradictory notions, namely, their widespread association with low-end jobs versus the high social status that is widely assigned to medical doctors. Thus, I capture the inconsistency in German public opinion and political attitudes towards immigration, as well as the heterogeneity of migrant groups. I verify these factors with qualitative empirical evidence giving this migration a "human face" (Favell et al., 2007) and highlight the significance of informal recognition for the successful integration of migrants in the workplace. My findings are an important contribution to an improved way of incorporating migrants – whether in medicine or other occupational fields, whether immigrating or already living in Germany.

8 References

Abbott, A. (1988). *The system of professions: an essay on the division of expert labor.* Chicago: University of Chicago Press.

Adler, G., & v. d. Knesebeck, J.-H. (2011). Ärztemangel und Ärztebedarf in Deutschland? Fragen an die Versorgungsforschung. *Bundesgesundheitsblatt, 54,* 228–237.

Allsop, J., Bourgeault, I. L., Evetts, J., Le Bianic, T., Jones, K., & Wrede, S. (2009). Encountering Globalization: Professional Groups in an International Context. *Current Sociology, 57*(4), 487-510. doi: 10.1177/0011392109104351

Allsop, J., & Mulcahy, L. (1998). Deconstructing and Reconstructing Professional Identity: Doctors' Responses to Complaints. In V. Olgiati, L. Orzack & M. Saks (Eds.), *Professions, Identity, And Order in Comparative Perspective* (pp. 123–148). Oñati: The International Institute for the Sociology of Law.

Bahna, M. (2012). Intra-EU Migration from Slovakia. *European Societies, 15*(3), 388-407. doi: 10.1080/14616696.2012.707669

BAMF. (2011). Anerkennung und Berufszugang für Ärzte und Fachärzte mit ausländischen Qualifikationen in Deutschland: Bundesministerium für Migration und Flüchtlinge (BAMF).

BAMF. (2013). Willkommens- und Anerkennungskultur. Handlungsempfehlungen und Praxisbeispiele. Abschlussbericht Runder Tisch "Aufnahmegesellschaft". Nürnberg: Bundesamt für Migration und Flüchtlinge (BAMF).

Bauder, H. (2003). "Brain Abuse", or the Devaluation of Immigrant Labour in Canada. *Antipode, 35*(4), 699-717.

Bauder, H. (2005). Institutional Capital and Labour Devaluation: The Non-Recognition of Foreign Credentials in Germany. *Journal of Economics, 2*(1), 75-93.

Beck, U. (1992). Risk society: towards a new modernity. London: Sage.

Becker, G. S. (1993). Human Capital. A Theoretical and Empirical Analysis with Special Reference to Education. Chicago and London: The University of Chicago Press.

Bernstein, J. H. (2000). The Professional Self-Evaluation of Migrant Physicians from the Former Soviet Union in Israel. *Journal of Immigrant Health, 2*(4).

Bidgood, E. (2013). Health Care Systems: Germany. Based on the 2001 Civitas Report by David Green and Benedict Irvine. Updated by Emily Clark (2012) and Elliot Bidgood (January 2013): Civitas.

Birsl, U. (2003). Deutschland. In W. Gieler (Ed.), *Handbuch der Ausländer- und Zuwanderungspolitik: von Afghanistan bis Zypern* (pp. 129-147). Münster [et al.]: Lit.

Black, R., Engbersen, G., Okólski, M., & Pantiru, C. (Eds.). (2010). *A continent moving west? EU enlargement and labour migration from Central and Eastern Europe.* Amsterdam: Amsterdam University Press.

Blitz, B. K. (2005). 'Brain circulation': the Spanish medical profession and international medical recruitment in the United Kingdom. *Journal of European Social Policy, 15*(4), 363-379. doi: 10.1177/0958928705057279

Bloor, G., & Dawson, P. (1994). Understanding Professional Culture in Organizational Context. *Organization Studies, 15*(2), 275-295. doi: 10.1177/017084069401500205

Blum, K., & Löffert, S. (2010). Ärztemangel im Krankenhaus - Ausmaß, Ursachen, Gegenmaßnahmen *Forschungsgutachten im Auftrag der Deutschen Krankenhausgesellschaft*: Deutsches Krankenhausinstitut.

Blum, K., Löffert, S., Offermanns, M., & Steffen, P. (2013). *Krankenhaus Barometer. Umfrage 2013*. Retrieved from http://www.dki.de/sites/default/files/downloads/krankenhaus_barometer_2013.pdf

Bogner, A., Littig, B., & Menz, W. (2014). *Interviews mit Experten: eine praxisorientierte Einführung*. Wiesbaden: Springer VS.

Bollinger, H., & Hohl, J. (1989). Auf dem Weg von der Profession zum Beruf. Zur Deprofessionalisierung des Ärzte-Standes. *Soziale Welt, 32*(4), 440-464.

Bölt, U., & Graf, T. (2012). 20 Jahre Krankenhausstatistik. Wiesbaden: Statistisches Bundesamt, Wirtschaft und Statistik.

Bonß, W., & Zinn, J. (2005). Erwartbarkeit, Glück und Vertrauen - Zum Wandel biographischer Sicherheitskonstruktionen in der Moderne. *Soziale Welt, 56*(2/3), 183-202. doi: 10.2307/40878492

Borchardt, K. (2006). Ärztemigration von und nach Deutschland. Theoretische und empirische Untersuchung unter besonderer Berücksichtigung der deutsch-polnischen Grenzregion Brandenburg. Baden-Baden: Nomos Verlag Gesellschaft.

Bourdieu, P. (1984). *Distinction. A social critique of the judgement of taste*. Cambridge: Harvard University Press.

Bourdieu, P. (2009). *Language and symbolic power*. Cambridge [et al.]: Polity Press.

Braun, M., & Arsene, C. (2009). The demographics of movers and stayers in the European Union. In E. Recchi & A. Favell (Eds.), *Pioneers of European integration: citizenship and mobility in the EU* (pp. 26-51). Cheltenham [et al.]: Edward Elgar.

Breckner, R. (2007). Case-oriented Comparative Approaches. The Biographical Perspective as Potential and Challenge in Migration Research. In K. Schittenhelm (Ed.), Concepts and Methods in Migration Research. Conference Reader. Retrieved from http://sowi-serv2.sowi.uni-due.de/cultural-capital/reader/Concepts-and-Methods.pdf.

Bryman, A. (2012). *Social research methods* (4th ed.). Oxford [et al.]: Oxford University Press.

Bundesärztekammer. (2006). Ärztemangel in Ostdeutschland. Beschlussprotokoll des 107. Deutschen Ärztetages vom 18.-21. Mai 2004 in Bremen. Retrieved 08/28/2015, from http://www.bundesaerztekammer.de/page.asp?his=0.2.23.2054.2090.2094

Bundesärztekammer. (2011). Ergebnisse der Ärztestatistik zum 31.12.2010. Diagramme und Tabellen. Retrieved 08/27/2015, 2011, from http://www.bundesaerztekammer.de/page.asp?his=0.3.9237

Bundesärztekammer. (2012). Ergebnisse der Ärztestatistik zum 31. Dezember 2011. Kein Widerspruch - Ärztemangel trotz steigender Arztzahlen. Retrieved 08/27/2015, from http://www.bundesaerztekammer.de/page.asp?his=0.3.10275

Bundesärztekammer. (2013a). Ergebnisse der Ärztestatistik zum 31. Dezember 2012. Alle Diagramme und Tabellen. Retrieved 08/28/2015, from http://www.bundesaerztekammer.de/downloads/Stat12Abbildungsteil.pdf

Bundesärztekammer. (2013b). Ergebnisse der Ärztestatistik zum 31. Dezember 2012. Kein Widerspruch - Ärztemangel trotz moderat steigender Arztzahlen. Retrieved 08/28/2015, from http://www.bundesaerztekammer.de/ueber-uns/aerztestatistik/aerztestatistik-der-vorjahre/aerztestatistik-2012/

Bundesärztekammer. (2014a). Ergebnisse der Ärztestatistik zum 31. Dezember 2013. Alle Diagramme und Tabellen. Retrieved 08/20/2015, from http://www.bundesaerztekammer.de/fileadmin/user_upload/downloads/Stat13AbbTab.pdf

Bundesärztekammer. (2014b). Ergebnisse der Ärztestatistik zum 31. Dezember 2013. Ärzteschaft in der Generationenfalle. Retrieved 08/28/2015, from http://www.bundesaerztekammer.de/page.asp?his=0.3.12002

Bundesärztekammer. (2014c). The Health Care System in Germany. Retrieved 08/27/2015, from http://www.bundesaerztekammer.de/page.asp?his=4.3571

Bundesärztekammer. (2015a). Ärztestatistik 2014: Etwas mehr und doch zu wenig. Retrieved 08/20/2015, from http://www.bundesaerztekammer.de/ueber-uns/aerztestatistik/aerztestatistik-2014/

Bundesärztekammer. (2015b). Ergebnisse der Ärztestatistik zum 31. Dezember 2014: Alle Diagramme und Tabellen. Retrieved 08/21/2015, from http://www.bundesaerztekammer.de/fileadmin/user_upload/downloads/pdf-Ordner/Statistik2014/Stat14AbbTab.pdf

Burrell, K. (2010). Staying, returning, working and living: key themes in current academic research undertaken in the UK on migration movements from Eastern Europe. *Social Identities: Journal for the Study of Race, Nation and Culture, 16*(3), 297-308. doi: 10.1080/13504630.2010.482401

Busse, R., & Riesberg, A. (2004). Health Care Systems in Transition. Germany: World Health Organisation.

bvmd. (2014). Konzeptpapier Zukunft und Weiterentwicklung des Medizinstudiums. In B. d. M. i. Deutschland (Ed.).

Carlson, S. (2013). Becoming a Mobile Student – a Processual Perspective on German Degree Student Mobility. *Population, Space and Place, 19*(2), 168-180. doi: 10.1002/psp.1749

Chapman, B. J., & Iredale, R. R. (1993). Immigrant Qualifications: Recognition and Relative Wage Outcomes. *The International Migration Review, 27*(2), 359-387. doi: 10.2307/2547129

Ciupijus, Z. (2011). Mobile Central Eastern Europeans in Britain: successful European Union citizens and disadvantaged labour migrants? *Work, Employment & Society, 25*(3), 540-550. doi: 10.1177/0950017011407962

Clark, K., & Drinkwater, S. (2008). The labour-market performance of recent migrants. *Oxford Review of Economic Policy, 24*(3), 495–516.

Collins, H. M. (1993). The Structure of Tacit Knowledge. *Social Research, 60*(1), 95-116.

Conradson, D., & Latham, A. (2005). Transnational urbanism: Attending to everyday practices and mobilities. *Journal of Ethnic and Migration Studies, 31*(2), 227-233. doi: 10.1080/1369183042000339891

Csedő, K. (2008). Negotiating Skills in the Global City: Hungarian and Romanian Professionals and Graduates in London. *Journal of Ethnic and Migration Studies, 34*(5), 803-823. doi: 10.1080/13691830802106093

Csedő, K. (2010). Markets and networks: channels towards the employment of Eastern European professionals and graduates in London. In R. Black, G. Engbersen & M. Okólski (Eds.), *A continent moving West? EU enlargement and labour migration from Central and Western Europe* (pp. 89-114). Amsterdam: Amsterdam University Press.

Currie, S. (2007). De-Skilled and Devalued: The Labour Market Experience of Polish Migrants in the UK Following EU Enlargement. *The International Journal of Comparative Labour Law and Industrial Relations, 23*(1), 83-116.

Cyrus, N. (2000). Mobile Migrationsmuster. Zuwanderung aus Polen in die Bundesrepublik Deutschland. *Berliner Debatte Initial, 11*(5/6), 95-103.

Cyrus, N. (2001). Schattenwirtschaft und Migration. Ethnologische Annäherungen an ein offenes Geheimnis. In F. Gesemann (Ed.), *Migration und Integration in Berlin. Wissenschaftliche Analysen und politische Perspektiven* (pp. 209-232). Opladen: Leske + Budrich.

Daheim, H. (1992). Zum Stand der Professionssoziologie. Rekonstruktion machttheoretischer Modelle der Profession. In B. Dewe, W. Ferchhoff & F.-O. Radtke (Eds.), *Erziehen als Profession. Zur Logik professionellen Handelns in pädagogischen Feldern* (pp. 21-35). Opladen: Leske + Budrich.

den Adel, M., Blauw, W., Dobson, J., Hoesch, K., & Salt, J. (2004). *Recruitment and the Migration of Foreign Workers in Health and Social Care.* Imis-Beiträge, (25). Osnabrück.

Dewe, B. (1996). Das Professionswissen von Weiterbildnern: Klientenbezug - Fachbezug. In A. Combe & W. Helsper (Eds.), *Pädagogische Professionalität. Untersuchungen zum Typus pädagogischen Handelns* (pp. 714-757). Frankfurt/M.: Suhrkamp.

Di Luzio, G. (2005). Professionalismus - eine Frage des Vertrauens? In M. Pfadenhauer (Ed.), *Professionelles Handeln* (pp. 69-85). Wiesbaden: VS Verlag für Sozialwissenschaften.

Dietz, B. (2002). East west migration patterns in an enlarging Europe: The German case. *Global Review of Ethnopolitics, 2*(1), 29-43. doi: 10.1080/14718800208405121

Dietz, B. (2007). Die Integration mittel- und osteuropäischer Zuwanderer in den deutschen Arbeitsmarkt. In M. Nowicka (Ed.), *Von Polen nach Deutschland. Die Arbeitsmigration und ihre Herausforderungen für Europa* (pp. 25-45). Bielefeld: transcript Verlag.

DKI, & medirandum. (2012). *Ärztestellenbarometer Herbst 2012.* Retrieved from https://www.dki.de/sites/default/files/downloads/aerztestellen_barometer_herbst_2012.pdf

Drinkwater, S., Eade, J., & Garapich, M. (2009). Poles Apart? EU Enlargement and the Labour Market Outcomes of Immigrants in the United Kingdom. *International Migration, 47*(1), 161-190.

Drinkwater, S., & Garapich, M. P. (2015). Migration Strategies of Polish Migrants: Do They Have Any at All? *Journal of Ethnic and Migration Studies*, 1-23. doi: 10.1080/1369183X.2015.1027180

Elsner, B., & Zimmermann, K. F. (2013). *10 Years After: EU Enlargement, Closed Borders, and Migration to Germany.* Discussion Paper Series, (7103). Bonn.

Engbersen, G., & Snel, E. (2013). Liquid migration. Dynamic and fluid patterns of post-accession migration flows. In B. Glorius, I. Grabowska-Lusinska & A. Kuvik (Eds.), *Mobility in Transition. Migration Patterns after EU enlargement* (pp. 21-40). Amsterdam: Amsterdam University Press.

Eraut, M. (2000). Non-formal learning and tacit knowledge in professional work. *British Journal of Educational Psychology, 70*, 113-136.

Fassmann, H., & Münz, R. (1994). European East-West Migration, 1945-1992. *International Migration Review, 28*(3), 520-538. doi: 10.2307/2546819
Favell, A. (2008a). Eurostars and Eurocities: free movement and mobility in an integrating Europe. Malden, Mass. [et al.]: Blackwell.
Favell, A. (2008b). The new face of East-West migration in Europe. *Journal of Ethnic and Migration Studies, 34*(5), 701–716.
Favell, A. (2013). The Changing Face of 'Integration' in a Mobile Europe. *Council For European Studies Newsletter, 43*(1), 53-58.
Favell, A., Feldblum, M., & Smith, M. P. (2007). The human face of global mobility: A research agenda. *Society, 44*(2), 15–25.
Favell, A., Feldblum, M., & Smith, M. P. (2008). The Human Face of Global Mobility: A Research Agenda. In M. P. Smith & A. Favell (Eds.), *The Human Face of Global Mobility: international highly skilled migration in Europe, North America and the Asia-Pacific*. New Brunswick and London: Transaction Publishers.
Fellmer, S. (2007). Was erleichtert, was hemmt die Zuwanderung polnischer Ärzte. Analyse ihrer Migrationsentscheidung und der relevanten deutschen Zuwanderungspolitik. *Zeitschrift für Arbeitsmarktforschung, 40*(1), 23–44.
Fellmer, S. (2008). *Germany Restricted the Freedom of Movement for Polish Citizens - But Does it Matter?* Across Fading Borders: The Challenges of East-West Migration in the EU. eumap.org, Osnabrück.
Fihel, A., Kaczmarczyk, P., & Okólski, M. (2006). Labour Mobility in the Enlarged European Union. International Migration from the EU8 countries. CMR Working Papers, (14/72). Warsaw.
Finotelli, C. (2014a). In the Name of Human Capital. The International Recruitment of Physicians in Germany and Spain. *Comparative Migration Studies, 2*(4), 493-517.
Finotelli, C. (2014b). The international recruitment of physicians and IT and engineering specialist in Germany and Spain: actors, processes and challenges. fieri Working Paper.
Fligstein, N. (2001). The architecture of markets: an economic sociology of twenty-first century capitalist societies. Princeton, NJ [et al.]: Princeton University Press.
Fox, J. E., Moroşanu, L., & Szilassy, E. (2012). The Racialization of the New European Migration to the UK. *Sociology, 46*(4), 680-695. doi: 10.1177/0038038511425558
Freidson, E. (1970). Profession of Medicine. A Study of the Sociology of Applied Knowledge. New York: Dodd, Mead & Company.
Galasińska, A., & Kozłowska, O. (2009). Discourses of a 'Normal Life' among Post-accession Migrants from Poland to Britain. After 2004. In K. Burrell (Ed.), *Polish migration to the UK in the 'new' European Union* (pp. 87-105). Farnham [et al.]: Ashgate.
García-Pérez, M. A., Amaya, C., & Otero, Á. (2007). Physicians' migration in Europe: an overview of the current situation. *Bmc Health Services Research, 7*(1), 201.
Gerhards, J., & Lengfeld, H. (2009). Europäisierte Chancengleichheit? *Berliner Journal für Soziologie, 19*(4), 627-652. doi: 10.1007/s11609-009-0111-2
Gerlinger, T. (2011). Versorgung in ländlichen Regionen. *Public Health Forum, 19*(70), 13.e11-13.e13.
Girard, E. R., & Bauder, H. (2007). Assimilation and Exclusion of Foreign Trained Engineers in Canada: Inside a Professional Regulatory Organization. *Antipode, 39*(1), 35-53.

Glinos, I. A., & Buchan, J. (2014). Health professionals crossing the EU's internal and external borders: a typology of health professional mobility and migration. In J. Buchan, M. Wismar, I. A. Glinos & J. Bremner (Eds.), *Health professional mobility in a changing Europe. New dynamics, mobile individuals and diverse responses* (pp. 129-151). Copenhagen: World Health Organization.

Glorius, B. (2007). Zeiträume der Migration: Migrations- und Integrationsverläufe polnischer Migranten in Leipzig vor dem Hintergrund individueller und struktureller Umbrüche. Migration und residentielle Mobilität: Chancen der Integration und Risiken der Segregation. Universität Bremen, MIGREMUS. Bremen.

Glorius, B., Grabowska-Lusinska, I., & Kuvik, A. (Eds.). (2013). *Mobility in Transition. Migration Patterns after EU enlargement*. Amsterdam: Amsterdam University Press.

Gottschall, K., & Schwarzkopf, M. (2010). Irreguläre Arbeit in Privathaushalten. Rechtliche und institutionelle Anreize zu irregulärer Arbeit in Privathaushalten in Deutschland. Bestandaufnahme und Lösungsansätze. Hans-Böckler-Stiftung. Arbeitspapier, (217). Düsseldorf.

Granovetter, M. (1985). Economic Action and Social Structure: The Problem of Embeddedness. *American Journal of Sociology, 91*(3), 481-510. doi: 10.2307/2780199

Grignon, M., Owusu, Y., & Sweetman, A. (2012). *The international migration of health professionals*. IZA Discussion Paper Series, (6517). Bonn.

Grigoleit, G. (2012). "In Deutschland muss man sich seine Position noch erkämpfen" - Hochqualifizierte Migrantinnen in Unternehmen im Technologiesektor. In I. Jungwirth, G. Grigoleit & A. Wolffram (Eds.), *Arbeitsmarktintegration hochqualifizierter Migrantinnen. Berufsverläufe in Naturwissenschaft und Technik* (pp. 25-33). Bonn, Berlin: Bundesministerium für Bildung und Forschung (BMBF).

Gustafson, P. (2002). Tourism and seasonal retirement migration. *Annals of Tourism Research, 29*(4), 899-918. doi: http://dx.doi.org/10.1016/S0160-7383(01)00084-6

Guth, J., & Gill, B. (2008). Motivations in east-west doctoral mobility: Revisiting the question of brain drain. *Journal of Ethnic and Migration Studies, 34*(5), 825-841. doi: 10.1080/13691830802106119

Hans, S. (2010). Assimilation oder Segregation? Anpassungsprozesse von Einwanderern in Deutschland. Wiesbaden: VS Verlag für Sozialwissenschaften.

Harris, A. (2011). In a moment of mismatch: overseas doctors' adjustments in new hospital environments. *Sociology of Health & Illness, 33*(2), 308-320. doi: 10.1111/j.1467-9566.2010.01307.x

Hass, H.-D., & Neumair, S.-M. (n.d.). Stadt. *Gabler Wirtschaftslexikon*. from http://wirtschaftslexikon.gabler.de/Archiv/9180/stadt-v9.html

Heckmann, F. (2003). From Ethnic Nation to Universalistic Immigrant Integration: Germany. In F. Heckmann & D. Schnapper (Eds.), *The integration of immigrants in European societies: national differences and trends of convergence; in memory of Hans Mahnig* (pp. 45-78). Stuttgart: Lucius & Lucius.

Heinen, M., & Pegels, A. (2006). Die Übergangsregelungen. Retrieved 08/27/2015, from http://www.bpb.de/gesellschaft/migration/dossier-migration/57427/uebergangsregelungen

Helfferich, C. (2011). Die Qualität qualitativer Daten: Manual für die Durchführung qualitativer Interviews (4th ed.). Wiesbaden: VS Verlag für Sozialwissenschaften.

Helmreich, R. L., & Merritt, A. C. (2008). Culture at work in aviation and medicine. National, organizational and professional influences. Hampshire: Ashgate Publishing Limited.

Herfs, P. G. P., Kater, L., & Haalboom, J. R. E. (2007). Non-EEA doctors in EEA countries: doctors or cleaners? *Medical Teacher, 29*(4), 383-389. doi: 10.1080/01421590701477399

Heru, A. (2005). Pink-collar medicine: Women and the future of medicine. *Gender Issues, 22*(1), 20-34. doi: 10.1007/s12147-005-0008-0

Hespeler, U. (2000). Zur Erteilung der Approbation an ausländische Ärzte. *Medizinrecht, 18*(7), 333-335.

Hillienhof, A., & Hibbeler, B. (2014). Nordrhein-Westfalen. Ärztekammern übernehmen Sprachprüfung, *Deutsches Ärzteblatt*.

Hoesch, K. (2003). „Green Card" für Ärzte? Von der „Ärzteschwemme" zum Ärztemangel im deutschen Gesundheitssektor. Imis-Beiträge, (22). IMIS, Osnabrück.

Hoesch, K. (2012). Migrant Britain, sustainable Germany: Explaining differences in the international migration of health professionals. COMPAS Working Paper, (12-99). COMPAS, Oxford.

Hönekopp, E. (1997). Labour Migration to Germany from Central and Eastern Europe - Old and New Trends. IAB Labour Market Research Topics, (23). IAB, Nürnberg.

Hughes, D. (1988). When nurse knows best: some aspects of nurse/doctor interaction in a casualty department. *Sociology of Health & Illness, 10*(1), 1-22. doi: 10.1111/1467-9566.ep11340102

Hughes, E. C. (1945). Dilemmas and Contradictions of Status. *American Journal of Sociology, 50*(5), 353-359.

Huijskens, E. G. W., Hooshiaran, A., Scherpbier, A., & Van Der Horst, F. (2010). Barriers and facilitating factors in the professional careers of international medical graduates. *Medical Education, 44*(8), 795–804.

Humphries, N., Bidwell, P., Tyrrell, E., Brugha, R., Thomas, S., & Normand, C. (2014). "I am a kind of stalemate". The experiences of non-EU doctors in Ireland. In J. Buchan, M. Wismar, I. A. Glinos & J. Bremner (Eds.), *Health professional mobility in a changing Europe. New dynamics, mobile individuals and diverse responses* (pp. 233-250). Copenhagen: World Health Organization.

Iredale, R. (1999). The Need to Import Skilled Personnel: Factors Favouring and Hindering its International Mobility. *International Migration, 37*(1), 89-123. doi: 10.1111/1468-2435.00067

Iredale, R. (2001). The Migration of Professionals: Theories and Typologies. *International Migration, 39*(5), 7-26. doi: 10.1111/1468-2435.00169

Ivancheva, M. (2007). Strawberry fields forever? Bulgarian and Romanian student workers in the UK. *Focaal, 49*, 110-117.

Jefferies, D., & Evetts, J. (2000). Approaches to the international recognition of professional qualifications in engineering and the sciences. *European Journal of Engineering Education, 25*(1), 99-107. doi: 10.1080/030437900308670

Jinks, C., Ong, B. N., & Paton, C. (2000). Mobile medics? The mobility of doctors in the European Economic Area. *Health Policy, 54*(1), 45-64. doi: http://dx.doi.org/10.1016/S0168-8510(00)00097-X

Joppke, C. (1999). Immigration and the nation-state: the United States, Germany, and Great Britain. Oxford [et al.]: Oxford University Press.

Junge, M. (2014). Scheitern in Moderne und Postmoderne. In R. John & A. Langhof (Eds.), *Scheitern - ein Desiderat der Moderne*. Wiesbaden: Springer Fachmedien Wiesbaden.

Jungwirth, I. (2008). The change of normative gender orders in the process of migration: a transnational perspective. Arbeitspapier, (48). Center for Interdisciplinary Research, Bielefeld.

Jungwirth, I. (2011). The change of normative gender orders in the course of migration: highly qualified migrant women in Germany. In M. Nowak & M. Nowosielski (Eds.), *(Post)transformational Migration. Inequalities, Welfare State and Horizontal Mobility* (Vol. 13, pp. 225-250). Frankfurt a.M. [et al.]: Peter Lang.

Jungwirth, I. (2012). Geographische Mobilität und beschränkte Möglichkeiten - Berufsverläufe hochqualifizierter Migrantinnen. In I. Jungwirth, G. Grigoleit & A. Wolffram (Eds.), *Arbeitsmarktintegration hochqualifizierter Migrantinnen. Berufsverläufe in Naturwissenschaft und Technik* (pp. 15-24). Bonn, Berlin: Bundesministerium für Bildung und Forschung (BMBF).

Kaczmarczyk, P. (2007). Arbeitskraftwanderung aus Polen - die Erwartungen vor und die Realität nach der EU-Osterweiterung. In M. Nowicka (Ed.), *Von Polen nach Deutschland und zurück. Die Arbeitsmigration und ihre Herausforderungen für Europa*. Bielefeld: Transcript Verlag.

Kaczmarczyk, P. (2011). Polen in Bewegung. Migration nach dem EU-Beitritt. *Osteuropa, 61*(5-6), 175-188.

Kämpfer, S. (2014). Migration und Lebenszufriedenheit. Eine theoriegeleitete empirische Analyse. Opladen [et al.]: Budrich UniPress.

Kelle, U., & Kluge, S. (2010). Vom Einzelfall zum Typus: Fallvergleich und Fallkontrastierung in der qualitativen Sozialforschung (2nd ed.). Wiesbaden: VS Verlag für Sozialwissenschaften.

King, R. (2002). Towards a new map of European migration. *International Journal of Population Geography, 8*(2), 89–106.

King, R., & Ruiz-Gelices, E. (2003). International student migration and the European 'Year Abroad': effects on European identity and subsequent migration behaviour. *International Journal of Population Geography, 9*(3), 229-252. doi: 10.1002/ijpg.280

King, R., Warnes, A. M., & Williams, A. M. (1998). International retirement migration in Europe. *International Journal of Population Geography, 4*(2), 91-111. doi: 10.1002/(SICI)1099-1220(199806)4:2<91::AID-IJPG97>3.0.CO;2-S

Klein, J. (2015). Migration of Central Eastern European Physicians to Germany: An Empirical Description of the Field. In M. Pilati, H. Sheikh, F. Sperotti & C. Tilly (Eds.), *How Global Migration Changes the Workforce Diversity Equation* (pp. 101-126). Cambridge: Cambridge Scholars Publishing.

Klenk, T., & Pieper, J. (2013). Accountability in a Privatized Welfare State: The Case of the German Hospital Market. *Administration & Society, 45*(3), 326-356. doi: 10.1177/0095399712451890

Kley, S. (2011). Explaining the Stages of Migration within a Life-course Framework. *European Sociological Review, 27*(4), 469-486. doi: 10.1093/esr/jcq020

Kofman, E. (2000). The invisibility of skilled female migrants and gender relations in studies of skilled migration in Europe. *International Journal of Population Geography, 6*(1), 45-59. doi: 10.1002/(sici)1099-1220(200001/02)6:1<45::aid-ijpg169>3.0.co;2-b

Kofman, E., Phizacklea, A., Raghuram, P., & Sales, R. (2000). *Gender and international migration in Europe: employment, welfare and politics*. London and New York: Routledge.

Kofman, E., & Raghuram, P. (2010). Skilled female migrants in the discourse of labour migration in Europe. In H. B. Stiftung (Ed.), Dossier Mobilty & Inclusion. Managing Labour Migration in Europe. (pp. 55-59). Berlin.

Kohli, M. (2007). The Institutionalization of the Life Course: Looking Back to Look Ahead. *Research in Human Development, 4*(3-4), 253-271. doi: 10.1080/15427600701663122

Kolb, H. (2006). *Internationale Mobilität von Hochqualifizierten - (k)ein Thema für die Migrationsforschung*. Neue Zuwanderergruppen in Deutschland. Vorträge der 7. Tagung des Arbeitskreises Migration – Integration – Minderheiten der Deutschen Gesellschaft für Demographie (DGD) in Zusammenarbeit mit dem Soziologischen Institut der Universität Erlangen in Erlangen am 25. November 2005, (Materialband 118, Materialien zur Bevölkerungswissenschaft). Bundesinstitut für Bevölkerungsforschung (BiB) Wiesbaden.

Kołodziejska, A., Makulec, A., & Schulecka, M. (2012). *Poland. Mobility of Health Professionals*. MoHProf National Report.

Kopetsch, T. (2009). The migration of doctors to and from Germany. *Journal of Public Health, 17*(1), 33-39. doi: 10.1007/s10389-008-0208-7

Kopetsch, T. (2010). Dem deutschen Gesundheitswesen gehen die Ärzte aus! Studie zur Altersstruktur- und Arztzahlentwicklung (pp. 146).

Koslowski, R. (2000). Migrants and Citizens. Demographic Change in the European State System. Ithaca and London: Cornell University Press.

Kovacheva, V., & Grewe, M. (2015a). Migrant Workers in the German Health Sector *Work --> Int. project, Background Report*.

Kovacheva, V., & Grewe, M. (2015b). Workplace integration of migrant health workers in Germany. Qualitative findings on experiences in two Hamburg hospitals. *WORK->INT project, National Research Report*.

Krisjane, Z., Berzins, M., & Apsite, E. (2013). Post-accession migration from the Baltic states. The case of Latvia. In B. Glorius, I. Grabowska-Lusinska & A. Kuvik (Eds.), *Mobility in Transition. Migration Patterns after EU enlargement* (pp. 85-109). Amsterdam: Amsterdam University Press.

Lam, A. (2000). Tacit Knowledge, Organizational Learning and Societal Institutions: An Integrated Framework. *Organization Studies, 21*(3), 487-513.

Lutz, H. (2007). "Die 24-Stunden-Polin" - Eine intersektionelle Analyse transnationaler Dienstleistungen. In C. Klinger, G.-A. Knapp & B. Sauer (Eds.), *Achsen der Ungleichheit. Zum Verhältnis von Klasse, Geschlecht und Ethnizität* (pp. 210-234). Frankfurt/New York: Campus Verlag.

Lutz, H., & Palenga-Möllenbeck, E. (2010). Care Work Migration in Germany: Semi-Compliance and Complicity. *Social Policy and Society, 9*(03), 419-430. doi: doi:10.1017/S1474746410000138

Maas, W. (2007). *Creating European citizens*. Lanham, Md. [et al.]: Rowman & Littlefield.

MacKenzie, R., & Forde, C. (2009). The rhetoric of the 'good worker' versus the realities of employers' use and the experiences of migrant workers. *Work, Employment & Society, 23*(1), 142-159. doi: 10.1177/0950017008099783

Martin, P. (2004). Germany: managing migration in the 21st century. In W. A. Cornelius, P. L. Martin & J. F. Hollifield (Eds.), *Controlling Immigration: A Global Perspective*. Stanford: Stanford University Press.

Massey, D. S., Arango, J., Hugo, G., Kouaouci, A., Pellegrino, A., & Taylor, J. E. (1993). Theories of International Migration: A Review and Appraisal. *Population and Development Review, 19*(3), 431-466.

Mau, S., & Verwiebe, R. (2010). *European societies: mapping structure and change.* Bristol [et al.]: Policy Press.

Merkens, H. (2009). Auswahlverfahren, Sampling, Fallkonstruktion. In U. Flick (Ed.), *Qualitative Sozialforschung*. Reinbek: Rowohlt-Taschenbuch-Verlag.

Meuser, M., & Nagel, U. (2009). Experteninterview und der Wandel der Wissensproduktion. In A. Bogner, B. Littig & W. Menz (Eds.), *Experteninterviews. Theorien, Methoden, Anwendungsfelder* (pp. 35-60). Wiesbaden: VS Verlag für Sozialwissenschaften.

Morse, J. M. (1994). *Critical issues in qualitative research methods*. Thousand Oaks, California [u.a.]: Sage Publications, Inc.

Moutafova, E. (2011). *Bulgaria. Mobility of Health Professionals*. MoHProf national report.

Mulholland, J., & Ryan, L. (2014). Doing the Business: Variegation, Opportunity and Intercultural Experience among intra-EU Highly Skilled Migrants. *International Migration, 52*(3), 55-68.

Münz, R. (1996). A continent of migration: European mass migration in the twentieth century. *Journal of Ethnic and Migration Studies, 22*(2), 201-226. doi: 10.1080/1369183x.1996.9976535

n.n. (2014). Einheitliche Sprachtests für ausländische Ärzte beschlossen. Retrieved 08/27/2015, from http://m.aerzteblatt.de/news/59190.htm

Nohl, A.-M. (2010). Von der Bildung zum kulturellen Kapital: Die Akkreditierung ausländischer Hochschulabschlüsse auf deutschen und kanadischen Arbeitsmärkten. In A.-M. Nohl, K. Schittenhelm, O. Schmidtke & A. Weiß (Eds.), *Kulturelles Kapital in der Migration. Hochqualifizierte Einwanderer und Einwanderinnen auf dem Arbeitsmarkt* (pp. 153-165). Wiesbaden: VS Verlag für Sozialwissenschaften.

Nohl, A.-M., Ofner, U. S., & Thomsen, S. (2010). Hochqualifizierte BildungsausländerInnen in Deutschland: Arbeitsmarkterfahrungen unter den Bedingungen formaler Gleichberechtigung. In A.-M. Nohl, K. Schittenhelm, O. Schmidtke & A. Weiß (Eds.), *Kulturelles Kapital in der Migration. Hochqualifizierte Einwanderer und Einwanderinnen auf dem Arbeitsmarkt* (pp. 67-82). Wiesbaden: VS Verlag für Sozialwissenschaften.

Nohl, A.-M., Schittenhelm, K., Schmidtke, O., & Weiß, A. (2010a). Zur Einführung: Migration, kulturelles Kapital und Statuspassagen in den Arbeitsmarkt. In A.-M. Nohl, K. Schittenhelm, O. Schmidtke & A. Weiß (Eds.), *Kulturelles Kapital in der Migration Hochqualifizierte Einwanderer und Einwanderinnen auf dem Arbeitsmarkt* (pp. 9–35). Wiesbaden: VS Verlag für Sozialwissenschaften.

Nohl, A.-M., Schittenhelm, K., Schmidtke, O., & Weiß, A. (2014). *Work in Transition. Cultural Capital and Highly Skilled Migrants' Passages into the Labour Market.* Toronto et al.: University of Toronto Press.

Nohl, A.-M., Schittenhelm, K., Schmidtke, O., & Weiß, A. (Eds.). (2010b). *Kulturelles Kapital in der Migration. Hochqualifizierte Einwanderer und Einwanderinnen auf dem Arbeitsmarkt.* Wiesbaden: VS Verlag für Sozialwissenschaften.

Nohl, A.-M., & Weiß, A. (2011). Beyond the German "Green Card". Migration of Highly Qualified Professionals. *Unikate, 40,* 91-97.

Nowicka, M. (2012). Deskilling in migration in transnational perspective. The case of recent Polish migration to the UK. COMCAD Arbeitspapiere - Working Papers, (112). Bielefeld.

Nowicka, M. (2014). Successful Earners and Failing Others: Transnational Orientation as Biographical Resource in the Context of Labor Migration. *International Migration, 52*(1), 74-86. doi: 10.1111/imig.12144

OECD. (2013). Zuwanderung ausländischer Arbeitskräfte: Deutschland (German version). OECD Publishing. Berlin.

Ognyanova, D., Young, R., Maier, C. B., & Busse, R. (2014). Why do health professionals leave Germany and what attracts foreigners? A qualitative study. In J. Buchan, M. Wismar, I. A. Glinos & J. Bremner (Eds.), *Health professional mobility in a changing Europe. New dynamics, mobile individuals and diverse responses* (pp. 203-232). Copenhagen: World Health Organization.

Padaigia, Z., Pukas, M., & Starkienie, L. (2014). Health professional migration in Lithuania: why they leave and what makes them stay. In J. Buchan, M. Wismar, I. A. Glinos & J. Bremner (Eds.), *Health professional mobility in a changing Europe. New dynamics, mobile individuals and diverse responses* (pp. 155-176). Copenhagen: World Health Organization.

Palenga-Möllenbeck, E. (2013a). Care Chains in Eastern and Central Europe: Male and Female Domestic Work at the Intersections of Gender, Class, and Ethnicity. *Journal of Immigrant & Refugee Studies, 11*(4), 364-383.

Palenga-Möllenbeck, E. (2013b). New maids – new butlers? Polish domestic workers in Germany and commodification of social reproductive work. *Equality, Diversity and Inclusion: An International Journal, 32*(6), 557 - 574.

Parsons, T., & Shils, E. A. (1967). *Toward a General Theory of Action.* Cambridge: Harvard University Press.

Parutis, V. (2014). "Economic Migrants" or "Middling Transnationals"? East European Migrants' Experiences of Work in the UK. *International Migration, 52*(1), 36-55. doi: 10.1111/j.1468-2435.2010.00677.x

Patton, M. Q. (2002). *Qualitative research and evaluation methods* (3rd ed.). Thousand Oaks, California [et al.]: Sage.

Pfadenhauer, M. (2003). Professionalität. Eine wissenssoziologische Rekonstruktion institutionalisierter Kompetenzdarstellungskompetenz. Opladen: Leske + Budrich.

Pietka, E., Clark, C., & Canton, N. (2013). 'I know that I have a university diploma and I'm working as a driver.' Explaining the EU post-enlargement movement of Polish highly skilled workers to Glasgow. In B. Glorius, I. Grabowska-Lusinska & A. Kuvik (Eds.), *Mobility in Transition. Migration Patterns after EU enlargement* (pp. 133-154). Amsterdam: Amsterdam University Press.

Piore, M. J. (1979). *Birds of Passage: Migrant Labor in Industrial Societies.* Cambridge: Cambridge University Press.

Polanyi, M. (1966). *The Tacit Dimension.* Garden City New York: Doubleday.

Presidency Conlusions Council of the EU. Lisbon European Council. 23 and 24 March (2000).

Przyborski, A., & Wohlrab-Sahr, M. (2009). *Qualitative Sozialforschung: ein Arbeitsbuch* (2nd ed.). München: Oldenbourg Wissenschaftsverlag.

Pullon, S. (2008). Competence, respect and trust: Key features of successful interprofessional nurse-doctor relationships. *Journal of Interprofessional Care, 22*(2), 133-147.

Recchi, E. (2008). From Migrants to Movers. Citizenship and Mobility in the European Union. In M. P. Smith & A. Favell (Eds.), *The Human Face of Global Mobility: international highly skilled migration in Europe, North America and the Asia-Pacific* (pp. 53-80). New Brunswick and London: Transaction Publishers.

Recchi, E., & Favell, A. (Eds.). (2009). *Pioneers of European integration: citizenship and mobility in the EU*. Cheltenham [et al.]: Edward Elgar.

Reiter, H. (2010). Context, Experience, Expectation, and Action — Towards an Empirically Grounded, General Model for Analyzing Biographical Uncertainty. *Forum Qualitative Social Research, 11*(1). http://www.qualitative-research.net/index.php/fqs/article/view/1422/2913

Ribeiro, J. S. (2008). Migration and occupational integration: foreign health professionals in Portugal. In E. Kuhlmann & M. Saks (Eds.), *Rethinking professional governance. International directions in health care* (pp. 201-216). Bristol: Policy Press.

Rohova, M. (2011). *Romania. Mobility of Health Professionals*. MoHProf national report.

Roig, E. (2014). Care Crisis: Welche Auswirkungen haben Migrationspolitiken auf Geschlechtergerechtigkeit? Heinrich Böll Stiftung. E-Paper. Berlin.

Rubin, H. J., & Rubin, I. S. (2012). *Qualitative interviewing: the art of hearing data* (3rd ed.). Thousand Oaks, California [et al.]: SAGE.

Ryan, L., Klekowski Von Koppenfels, A., & Mulholland, J. O. N. (2015). 'The distance between us': a comparative examination of the technical, spatial and temporal dimensions of the transnational social relationships of highly skilled migrants. *Global Networks, 15*(2), 198-216. doi: 10.1111/glob.12054

Ryan, L., Sales, R., Tilki, M., & Siara, B. (2008). Social networks, social support and social capital: The experiences of recent Polish migrants in London. *Sociology-the Journal of the British Sociological Association, 42*(4), 672-690. doi: 10.1177/0038038508091622

Salaff, J., & Greve, A. (2003). Gendered Structural Barriers to Job Attainment for Skilled Chinese Emigrants in Canada. *International Journal of Population Geography, 9*, 443–456.

Saldaña, J. (2013). *The coding manual for qualitative researchers* (2nd ed.). Los Angeles [et al.]: Sage Publications.

Sander, K. (2009). Profession und Geschlecht im Krankenhaus: soziale Praxis der Zusammenarbeit von Pflege und Medizin. Konstanz: UVK-Verl.-Ges.

Santacreu, O., Baldoni, E., & Albert, M. C. (2009). Deciding to move: migration projects in an integrating Europe. In E. Recchi & A. Favell (Eds.), *Pioneers of European Integration. Citizenship and Mobility in the EU* (pp. 52-71). Cheltenham UK, Northampton, USA: Edward Elgar.

Schiller, M. (2010). Der Berufszugang ausländischer Ärzte. Eine systematische Darstellung der Approbationsvoraussetzungen in Fällen mit Auslandsbezug unter Berücksichtigung der aktuellen Rechtsprechung. *Medizinrecht, 28*(2), 79-86.

Scott, W. R. (2008). Lords of the Dance: Professionals as Institutional Agents. *Organization Studies, 29*(2), 219-238. doi: 10.1177/0170840607088151

Shuval, J. T. (2000). The Reconstruction of Professional Identity Among Immigrant Physicians in Three Societies. *Journal of Immigrant Health, 2*(4), 191-202. doi: 10.1023/a:1009588229071

Simon, M. (2012). Beschäftigte und Beschäftigungsstrukturen in Pflegeberufen. Eine Analyse der Jahre 1999 bis 2009. Studie für den deutschen Pflegerat. Hannover: Fachhochschule Hannover.

Sporton, D. (2013). 'They Control My Life': the Role of Local Recruitment Agencies in East European Migration to the UK. *Population Space and Place, 19*(5), 443-458. doi: 10.1002/psp.1732

Srur, N. (2010). Berufliche Integrationsförderung für immigrierte ÄrztInnen – Good Practice-Ansätze und die Entwicklung neuer Integrationsstrategien in Deutschland und Großbritannien. In A.-M. Nohl, K. Schittenhelm, O. Schmidtke & A. Weiß (Eds.), *Kulturelles Kapital in der Migration Hochqualifizierte Einwanderer und Einwanderinnen auf dem Arbeitsmarkt* (pp. 166–179). Wiesbaden: VS Verlag für Sozialwissenschaften.

Stein, L. I. (1967). The Doctor-Nurse Game. *Archives of General Psychiatry, 16*(6), 699-703.

Stein, L. I., Watts, D. T., & Howell, T. (1990). The doctor-nurse game revisited. *The New England Journal of Medicine, 322*(8), 546-549.

Strauss, A. L., & Corbin, J. M. (1991). *Basics of qualitative research: grounded theory procedures and techniques* (3rd ed.). Newbury Park, California [et al.]: Sage.

SVR. (2011). Migrationsland 2011. Jahresgutachten 2011 mit Migrationsbarometer. Berlin: Sachverständigenrat deutscher Stiftungen für Integration und Migration.

SVR. (2013). Erfolgsfall Europa? Folgen und Herausforderungen der EU-Freizügigkeit für Deutschland. Jahresgutachten 2013 mit Migrationsbarometer. Berlin: Sachverständigenrat deutscher Stiftungen für Integration und Migration.

Sweet, S. J., & Norman, I. J. (1995). The nurse-doctor relationship: a selective literature review. *Journal of Advanced Nursing, 22*(1), 165-170. doi: 10.1046/j.1365-2648.1995.22010165.x

Thränhardt, D. (1996). European migration from east to west: Present patterns and future directions. *Journal of Ethnic and Migration Studies, 22*(2), 227-242. doi: 10.1080/1369183x.1996.9976536

Thränhardt, D. (2002). Include or exclude: Discourses on immigration in Germany. *Journal of International Migration and Integration / Revue de l'integration et de la migration internationale, 3*(3-4), 345-362. doi: 10.1007/s12134-002-1019-2

Tietze, K. (2008). Migration von Hochqualifizierten im Kontext der Entwicklung der Einwanderungskonzepte deutscher Parteien. In U. Hunger, C. Aybek, A. Ette & I. Michalowski (Eds.), *Migrations- und Integrationsprozesse in Europa* (pp. 35-50): VS Verlag für Sozialwissenschaften.

Tjadens, F., Eckert, J., & Weilandt, C. (2012). Mobility of Health Professionals. Health systems, working conditions, patterns of health workers' mobility and implications for policy makers. WIAD - Scientific Institute of the Medical Association of German Doctors. Bonn.

Toader, E. (2012). Current Opinions of Doctors and Decisional Factors on the Migration of the Romanian Physicians: A Study of Several Mass-Media Statements. *Revista De Cercetare Si Interventie Sociala, 37*, 144-161.

Trevena, P. (2013). Why do highly educated migrants go for low-skilled jobs? A case study of Polish graduates working in London. In B. Glorius, I. Grabowska-Lusinska & A. Kuvik (Eds.), *Mobility in Transition. Migration Patterns after EU enlargement* (pp. 169-190). Amsterdam: Amsterdam University Press.

Tuffs, A. (2003). German doctors shun eastern states. *British Medical Journal, 327*(7421), 949.

Ulbricht, C. (2014). *Welcome (back) to Germany! The return of the guest-worker and its implications.* COMCAD Arbeitspapiere - Working Papers, (124). COMCAD, Bielefeld.

Ullah, A. A. (2010). Rationalizing Migration Decisions. Labour Migrants in East and South-East Asia. Farnham et al.: Ashgate.

Vandenbrande, T., Coppin, L., van der Hallen, P., Ester, P., Fourage, D., Fasang, A., . Schömann, K. (2006). Mobility in Europe. Analysis of the 2005 Eurobarometer survey on geographical and labour market mobility *European Foundation for the Improvement of Living and Working Conditions.* Dublin.

Verwiebe, R. (2004). Transnationale Mobilität innerhalb Europas: eine Studie zu den sozialstrukturellen Effekten der Europäisierung. Berlin: ed. sigma.

Verwiebe, R., Wiesböck, L., & Teitzer, R. (2014). New forms of intra-European migration, labour market dynamics and social inequality in Europe. *Migration Letters, 11*(2), 125-136.

Vysotskaya, V. (2011). Who goes? Who stays? Who returns? Migration journeys of highly skilled workers from Russia to Germany and back home. Frankfurt am Main: Lang.

Wagner, M., Fiałkowska, K., Piechowska, M., & Łukowski, W. (2013). Deutsches Waschpulver und polnische Wirtschaft. Die Lebenswelt polnischer Saisonarbeiter. Ethnographische Beobachtungen. Bielefeld: transcript Verlag.

Wallace, C., & Stola, D. (Eds.). (2001). *Patterns of Migration in Central Europe.* Basingstoke et al.: Palgrave Macmillan.

Weiß, A. (2005). The Transnationalization of Social Inequality: Conceptualizing Social Positions on a World Scale. *Current Sociology, 53*(4), 707-728. doi: 10.1177/0011392105052722

Weiß, A. (2010). Die Erfahrung rechtlicher Exklusion. Hochqualifizierte MigrantInnen und das Ausländerrecht. In A.-M. Nohl, K. Schittenhelm, O. Schmidtke & A. Weiß (Eds.), *Kulturelles Kapital in der Migration. Hochqualifizierte Einwanderer und Einwanderinnen auf dem Arbeitsmarkt* (pp. 123-137). Wiesbaden: VS Verlag für Sozialwissenschaften.

White, A., & Ryan, L. (2008). Polish 'Temporary' Migration: The Formation and Significance of Social Networks. *Europe-Asia Studies, 60*(9), 1467-1502.

Wingens, M., De Valk, H., Windzio, M., & Aybek, C. (2011). The Sociological Life Course Approach and Research on Migration and Integration. In M. Wingens, M. Windzio, H. De Valk & C. Aybek (Eds.), *A Life-Course Perspective on Migration and Integration* (pp. 1-13). Heidelberg, London, New York: Springer.

Wismar, M., Maier, C. B., Glinos, I. A., Dussault, G., & Figueras, J. (2011). *Health Professional Mobility and Health Systems. Evidence from 17 European Countries.* Copenhagen: World Health Organization.

Wissenschaftsrat. (2014). Empfehlungen zur Weiterentwicklung des Medizinstudiums in Deutschland auf Grundlage einer Bestandsaufnahme der humanmedizinischen Modellstudiengänge. In D. Wissenschaftsrat (Ed.). Dresden.

Witzel, A. (1982). Verfahren der qualitativen Sozialforschung. Überblick und Alternativen. Frankfurt am Main: Campus-Verlag.

Witzel, A., & Reiter, H. (2012). *The problem-centred interview.* Los Angeles [et al.]: Sage.

Wolanik Boström, K., & Öhlander, M. (2011). A Doctor's Life-story: On Professional Mobility, Occupational Sub-cultures and Personal Gains. In J. Isański & P. Luczys (Eds.), *Selling One's Favourtie Piano to Emigrate: Mobility Patterns in Central Europe at the Beginning of the 21st Century* (pp. 205-222). Newcastle upon Tyne: Cambridge Scholars Publishing.

Wolanik Boström, K., & Öhlander, M. (2012). *A troubled elite? Stories about migration and establishing professionalism as a Polish doctor in Sweden.* COMCAD Arbeitspapiere - Working Papers, (110). COMCAD, Bielefeld.

Yamamura, S. (2009). „Brain Waste" ausländischer Ärztinnen und Ärzte in Deutschland. *Wirtschaftsdienst, 89*(3), 196–201.

Zinn, J. O. (2004). Health, Risk and Uncertainty in the Life Course: A Typology of Biographical Certainty Constructions. *Social Theory & Health, 2,* 199–221.

Zinn, J. O. (2010). Biography, Risk and Uncertainty - Is there Common Ground for Biographical Research and Risk Research? *Forum: Qualitative Social Research, 11*(1). http://www.qualitative-research.net/index.php/fqs/article/view/1512/3030

9 Attachment

i. Interview guide of the expert interviews[251]

I. INTRODUCTION

  1. To start with, would you please tell me something about your position and your tasks here in this hospital?

II. START

  2. Why is it that you employ foreign/CEE physicians here in your hospital?
      a. Since when has that been the case?

III. RECRUITMENT

  3. I am particularly interested in the recruitment of CEE physicians. Would you please describe the ways in which you recruit these physicians and how the personnel selection procedure takes place?
      a. Does your hospital actively recruit foreign physicians? How is this recruitment pursued?
      b. Which job requirements do you apply?

  4. How does the recruitment procedure of these physicians take place?
      a. What is the formal procedure?
      b. Which bureaucratic steps have to be taken?

  5. How would you describe the physicians' initial phase in the hospital?
      a. Is there any kind of support? Please describe this support.
      b. **If not:** Why not – is that a conscious decision?

  6. Why do you employ foreign physicians?
      • If not already answered under 2.

---

[251] Both the expert interviews and the problem centered interviews were conducted in German. I subsequently translated the interview guides into English for the publication of the thesis.

IV.   COLLABORATION

   7.   Which experiences did you have with these physicians so far?
        a.   What challenges or problems do you encounter?
        b.   Are there differences between physicians from different countries?

   8.   How do you see the collaboration with colleagues?
        a.   How would you describe the work atmosphere?
        b.   Which difficulties and challenges occur during the daily routine?
        c.   Are there differences between physicians of different origin?

   9.   How do you assess the contact between foreign physicians and patients?

V.   HUMAN RESOURCE STRATEGIES (these questions were only posed to the HR managers, and not to the medical directors)

   10. How is the work time for physicians organised in this hospital?
        a.   Do you think the work time satisfies the needs of the physicians?
        b.   Do you think work time is equally and fairly allocated between physicians? Are there any particular advantages or disadvantages with this procedure?

   11. Which kind of support does your hospital provide for physicians with family/children?
        c.   Do they make use of it? Who uses it?
        d.   *If not*: Why? Is that a conscious decision?

   12. How is the remuneration of physicians structured?
        e.   Do you think the remuneration is fair?
        f.   **In case of basis for negotiation:** Does that lead to advantages or disadvantages? For whom?

VI.   SHORTAGE OF PHYSICIANS

   13. You mentioned the shortage of physicians in Germany/A shortage of physicians in Germany is widely discussed. What, do you think, are the reasons for this shortage and how could this be solved in the future?

14. It is often written that this shortage of physicians in Germany further increases vis-à-vis the general feminisation of medicine. What do you think about that?
    a. Do you observe such a feminisation in your hospital, too? To which specialisations does this apply?
    b. Does this development also apply to the physicians from CEE?

15. "Generation y", the generation of those who would sacrifice a career to a better "work-life-balance" is often discussed. Do you observe this phenomenon in this hospital and what does this imply with regard to the shortage of physicians in Germany?
    a. *If yes:* Are there differences between physicians of different origin?
    b. How do you respond to this development?

VII. TAKING STOCK

16. In summary, what is your perception on the international medical profession in this hospital?
    a. What has developed/changed in a positive or negative way?
    b. Regarding the future, what would be a good solution for the recruitment of foreign physicians in this hospital?

17. You mentioned a few/several difficulties with regard to the employment of foreign physicians. How do you think this can the situation can be improved?

OR

You describe the employment of foreign physicians in your hospital as unproblematic. Do you, nevertheless, have suggestions for what can be done better or differently?

ii. Interview guide of the problem-centred interviews

I. MIGRATION DECISION

1. Let's start with your professional career. Please tell me why you decided to study medicine. What were the separate steps of your training and what led you to finally take up your position in this hospital?
   a. What were your reasons for working here in this hospital? Why did you apply for this position? Why did you opt for this hospital?
   c. Which ideas/expectations did you associate with this step?
   d. How did you find out about this position?

2. What were the different steps of the application process?
   a. How complex was the application process?
   b. What help or support did you have?
   c. How satisfied have you been with the provided information and support?
   d. How did you experience the bureaucratic expense?

II. INITIAL PHASE

3. Do you still remember the early period when you began working in this hospital? How did you feel in this situation?
   a. What was new for you or unusual?
   b. Which potential difficulties did you struggle with?

4. How did that go in your initial phase? How did your integration into the hospital go?
   a. How did you learn about the procedures, the organization of work etc.?
   b. Would you have wished for more support with certain aspects?

III. COOPERATION and INTERACTION

5. How would you describe your cooperation with your colleagues?
   a. Are you familiar with this kind of cooperation?
   b. Do you receive support from your colleagues?
   c. Do you receive support from your superior?
   d. (Do you feel respected/accepted by your colleagues?)

6. How is your relationship with your colleagues outside of work?
   a. Did you, as a new physician, quickly connect with your colleagues?
   b. Do you spend your breaks together?
   c. (Do you maintain private contact with your colleagues?)
      - With whom?
      - How would you describe this relationship?

7. How about other hospital staff? How do you experience the collaboration between physicians on the one hand, and nurses on the other hand, in this hospital?
   a. Are you familiar with this kind of collaboration?
   b. How would you describe your contact with the nurses?
   c. (Do you feel accepted/respected by the nurses?)

8. How would you describe your relationship to the other (administrative) hospital staff?

9. What experiences have you had when interacting with patients?
   a. How would you describe your contact with patients?
   b. How do patients respond to you?
   c. What difficulties or challenges do you encounter when interacting with patients?
   d. How would you describe your conversations with patients and relatives?
   e. Were there any special incidents that you would like to tell me about?

10. Do you think your work is adequately appreciated?
    a. What makes you feel this way?

IV. WORKING CONDITIONS

11. What do you think about the working conditions?
    a. How do you experience would you describe your tasks and work load?
       - How do you organise your specialist training during your routine work requirements? Do you have sufficient opportunities/time for your residency?
    b. How are working times organised?
       - How flexible are you in determining work time and holidays?
       - How compatible are work and private life for you?

c. What is the procedure for remuneration?
- Do you think that you are paid adequately?
- Are there differences with regard to payment?
- Do you think your pay is appropriate and fair?

12. In some professional fields there are still inequalities in how men and women are treated. Is this the case in the medical profession?
  a. How is it in this hospital – does everyone have the same conditions and opportunities?
  b. Are the positions of senior and head physicians held more by women or men?
  c. *Potentially:* What could be the reasons for that?

V.   ESTABLISHMENT

13. How do you evaluate your current situation in this hospital? Do you feel like you have settled in by now?
  a. What makes you feel this way?
  b. What is easier or still difficult for you?

14. The German health care system is very complicated and difficult to understand for both patients and physicians. Are you familiar with the German health care system?
  a. *Potentially*: Why not?
  b. Would that be easier for you in your home country?

15. To what extent do you feel that the hospital administration recognises and considers your needs and interests in this hospital?
  a. Is there an organised representation of interests on the part of the physicians towards clinic management?
  b. Are you a member of a medical representation? *Potentially:* Why (not)? What are your expectations from this membership?
  c. Would you do that differently in your home country? Why?

VI. OPPORTUNITIES FOR ADVANCEMENT

16. How would you describe your professional goals?
  a. Do you receive support for these goals here on-site? In which form?

b. How do you estimate your professional advancement in this hospital? Do you think you can achieve your goals here?

c. Do you aim at the position of head physician? *Potentially:* Why not?

VII. TAKING STOCK/FUTURE

17. In retrospect, how do you see your decision to come here?
    a. Would you make the same decision again?
    b. Would you recommend your friends to do the same?
    c. Have your expectations been met?

18. When you reflect on your initial motivation to become a physician, what is your opinion on this given what you now know?

19. Where do you see yourself in 10-15 years?

iii.   Demographic questionnaire

Name:

Hospital:

Year of birth: Place of birth:

Citizenship: Gender:

Marital status (if applicable, citizenship of partner):

Children (yes/no):

Place of residence (if commuting, please indicate both places):

In Germany since (month/year):

Place of medical studies (city, country):

Place of specialist training (city, country):

Specialist since: /expected in:

Specialisation:

Current position:

Working in this hospital since:

Did you work in another hospital in Germany before?

If so, please give the start date and end date:

(   ) Yes, I agree to be interviewed.

You can contact me via (telephone/email):

iv. Transcription rules

- Length of noticeably long breaks flagged with counted seconds in parentheses, e.g. (5)

- Laughter:
    - Short outburst of laughter: @(.)@
    - Length of long laughter flagged with counted seconds: e.g. @(3)@
    - Laughing while speaking: e.g. @I totally misunderstood!@

- Interruptions/speaking at the same time flagged with brackets: e.g.
  Interviewer: When did you start working [in this hospital?
  IP00:   [I first came here in 2010.

- Broken off words flagged with hyphen: e.g. hospi-

- Broken off sentences flagged with: …

- Incomprehensible text passages:
    - Entirely incomprehensible: (?)
    - Insecure whether understood correctly flagged with parentheses: e.g. (hospital)

- Anonymization flagged with brackets:
    - Description: e.g. [home country] instead of Poland, [native language] instead of [Polish]

- Noticeably loud pronunciation flagged with underscore: e.g. really difficult

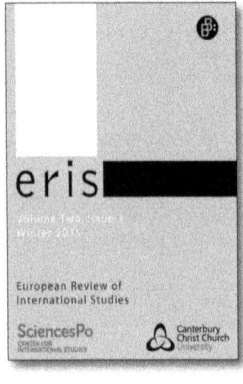
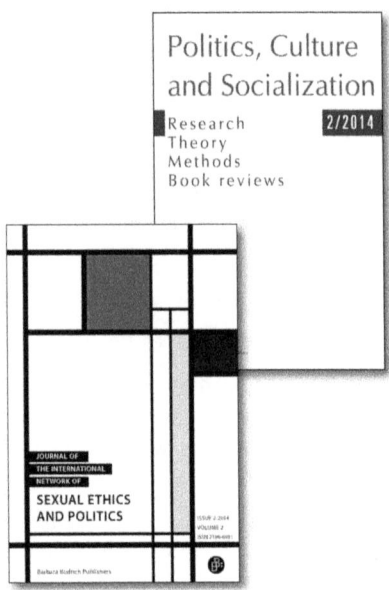

CPSIA information can be obtained
at www.ICGtesting.com
Printed in the USA
LVHW02s2349070118
562082LV00001B/4/P